# Type 2 diabetes mea[l]

# beginners

30-day Easy-to-make recipes to lower blood sugar for newly-diagnosed diabetics and advanced users. Rejuvenate and manage your body on healthy living

## Kenzie R. Cox

# Copyright

# Table of Contents

# 30-Day Diabetic Meal Plan

## Day 1

## Breakfast

Honey Garlic pork chops

Prep Time: 10 mins
Cook Time: 15 mins
Total Time: 25 mins
Servings: 6
Yield: 6 servings
Ingredients
- 2 tablespoons low-sodium soy sauce
- 6 (4 ounce) (1-inch thick) pork chops
- ½ cup ketchup
- 2 cloves garlic, crushed
- 2 ⅔ tablespoons honey

Instructions
1. Gather all the ingredients together and preheat the grill at a medium heat and give the grate a ⬚uick oiling.
2. To prepare a glaze, combine honey, ketchup, soy sauce, and garlic in a basin.
3. On the hot grill, sear the pork chops on both sides. As the chops cook, lightly brush the glaze over each side. Grill the chops for 7 to 9 minutes per side or until the middle is no longer pink. The internal temperature should be 145°F (63°C) using an instant-read thermometer.
4. Serve it hot and enjoy!

## Lunch

Super Crispy Chicken Wings

Servings: 12
Preparation Time: 5 Minutes
Cooking Time: 25 Minutes
Total Time: 30 Minutes
Ingredients
- 1 tablespoon (14.5g) baking powder
- 2 lb (907g) chicken wings

Instructions
- Utilizing paper towels, pat dry the chicken wings.
- Add wings and baking powder to a large basin. Turn the wings in the baking powder until it is well distributed.
- If using an air fryer, arrange the wings in a single layer in the basket, ensuring sure that none of them contact or overlap. If your air fryer is not big enough, you might need to cook in two batches. Before adding the wings, spray the bottom of your air fryer basket with cooking oil spray if it is not nonstick. Since the majority of air fryer baskets, I've seen are nonstick, oil spray is not required. Pre-heat your air fryer by setting the temperature to 400°F (204°C). Put the wings in after it reaches the proper temperature, and cook them for about 20 minutes, flipping them halfway through. Cook the wings for a further five minutes after the initial 20 minutes, or until the desired crispiness is reached.
- To begin cooking, preheat the oven to 250°F (121°C). Use foil to cover a sizable baking sheet. If the surface is not nonstick, place a cooling wire rack on top and spray cooking oil spray on it. On the cooling rack, arrange the wings in a single layer, taking care to avoid touching or overlapping any of them. In the lowest part of the oven, bake for 30 minutes. Turn up the oven's heat to 425°F (218°C). Re-place the wings in the oven, this time in the top center position. Bake wings for 50 minutes, or until desired crispiness is achieved.

# Dinner

## Carrot and Apple Salad

Preparation Time: 10 Minutes
Total Time: 10 Minutes
Servings: 6
Ingredients

### For the Salad:

- ¼ cup purple or sweet onion, finely diced
- 4 medium carrots, coarsely grated
- ¾ cup craisins, dried cranberries
- 1 apple, dice

### For the Dressing:

- 1/8 teaspoon sea salt, or to taste
- ½ cup mayonnaise, real mayo or vegenaise
- ½ tablespoon sugar
- Pinch of black pepper, freshly ground
- 2 teaspoon lemon juice

### Instructions

- Take a small basin, add 2 teaspoon of lemon juice, ½ cup mayo, pinch of pepper and salt, ½ tablespoon of sugar and mix together.
- Use a food processor to ⊡uickly coarsely grate the carrots, then transfer them to a sizable mixing basin. Apples and onions should be coarsely diced before being added to the bowl with the craisins.
- When the salad is ready to be served, toss everything together and add the salad dressing to taste.
- Enjoy your meal!

# Day 2

## Breakfast

### Banana Bread

Preparation Time: 10 Minutes
Cooking Time: 60 Minutes
Total Time: 70 Minutes
Servings: 8-10
Yield: 1 Loaf
Ingredients
- ½ teaspoon baking soda (not baking powder)
- 1 teaspoon vanilla extract
- 1/3 cup (76g) butter, unsalted or salted, melted
- 1 pinch salt
- 2 to 3 medium (7" to 7-7/8" long very ripe bananas, peeled (about 1 ¼ to 1 ½ cups mashed)
- 1 ½ cups (205g) all-purpose flour
- 1 large egg, beaten
- 3/4 cup (150g) sugar (1/2 cup if you would like it less sweet, 1 cup if sweeter)

Instructions
- Butter a loaf pan that measure 8 by 4 inches and preheat the oven to 350°F
- Use a fork to thoroughly mash the ripe bananas in a mixing dish. The mashed bananas are combined with the melted butter.
- Add the salt and baking soda together. Add vanilla essence, sugar, and one egg that has been beaten. Add flour and stir.
- Fill the loaf pan you have prepared with the batter. Bake at 350°F for 55 to 65 minutes, or until a wooden skewer or toothpick inserted into the center of the cake comes out clean. In contrast to moist batter streaks, a few dry crumbs are acceptable. Loosely tent the loaf with foil and bake it for

an additional few minute if the exterior of the loaf is browned but the inside is still damp.
- Take out of the oven, then let cool in the pan for a while. When ready to serve, take the banana bread out of the pan and let it cool fully. Slice, then dish. (Using a bread knife makes it easier to cut slices that won't crumble). The banana bread will keep for four days at room temperature if it is properly wrapped. The bread can be frozen or refrigerated for prolonged storage for up to 5 days.

## Lunch

## Chicken Noodles Soup

Preparation Time: 20 Minutes
Cooking Time: 20 Minutes
Total Time: 40 Minutes
Servings: 8
Ingredients
- 1 clove garlic, minced
- 1/8 teaspoon dried sage
- 1 batch homemade egg noodles, or 5 cups dry egg noodles, farfalle or other bite-size pasta
- 2 ribs celery, diced
- 1 teaspoon Better than Bouillon chicken base (or more, as needed) , or chicken bouillon granules
- 10 cups chicken stock
- 1/8 teaspoon crushed red pepper flakes
- ½ teaspoon freshly ground black pepper, to taste
- 3 cups rotisserie chicken
- 1 teaspoon salt, to taste
- 1/2 Tablespoon butter
- 3-4 large carrots diced
- 1/8 teaspoon dried rosemary, or more, to taste

Instructions

- Over medium-high heat, add diced celery, butter, and carrots to a sizable stockpot. 3 minutes of sauteing. Cook for 30 more seconds after adding the garlic.
- Add chicken stock and season the soup with salt, pepper, crushed red pepper, rosemary, sage, and crushed red pepper before tasting it. When necessary, taste and add "better than bullion" chicken bouillon cubes or granules.
- Boil the broth then add the noodles and cook them just until they are al dente, using either dry store-bought pasta or uncooked homemade egg noodles.
- Be careful not to overcook store-bought noodles if using them! Once they are just barely soft, turn off the heat. You don't want the noodles to become mushy since they will continue to cook once the heat is turned off.
- Chicken from the rotisserie chicken should be added. Once more tasting the soup, adjust the seasoning as desired.
- Depending on how fresh your chicken was, keep leftovers in an airtight jar in the fridge for 4-5 days.

## Dinner

### Lemon Pepper Chicken

Preparation Time: 10 Minutes
Cooking Time: 20 Minutes
Total Time: 30 Minutes
Serving: 1
Ingredients
- 2 boneless skinless chicken breasts (about 1.3 lbs. total)
- 2 Tbsp all-purpose flour
- 1 Tbsp lemon pepper seasoning
- 1 Tbsp cooking oil
- 1 clove garlic, minced
- 1/2 cup chicken broth
- 1 Tbsp butter
- 1 tsp lemon juice
- 1 Tbsp chopped fresh parsley (optional)

- 1/8 tsp freshly cracked black pepper

Instructions
- Use a sharp knife to carefully fillet the chicken breasts into two thinner peices (or use thin-cut chicken breasts).
- Combine the flour and lemon pepper seasoning in a bowl. Sprinkle the mixture over both sides of the chicken breast pieces and then rub it in until the chicken is fully coated.
- Heat the cooking oil in a large skillet over medium. When the skillet and oil are very hot, add the chicken and cook on each side until golden brown (about 5 minutes per side). Remove the cooked chicken to a clean plate and cover to keep warm.
- Add the butter and minced garlic to the skillet and sauté for about one minute.
- Add the chicken broth to the skillet and whisk to dissolve all the browned bits from the bottom of the skillet. Add the lemon juice and allow the sauce to simmer in the skillet for 3-5 minutes, or until it has reduced slightly. Taste the sauce and add salt if needed (I did not add any).
- Finally, return the chicken to the skillet and spoon the sauce over top. Allow the chicken to heat through. Season with a little freshly cracked pepper and fresh chopped parsley (optional), then serve.

# Day 3

## Breakfast

### Coconut Milk Porridge

Preparation Time: 5 Minutes
Cooking Time: 10 Minutes
Total Time: 15 Minutes
Servings: 2
Ingredients
- 1 cup oats
- 2 cups water
- ½ - 1 cup coconut milk
- ½ tsp cinnamon
- 1 tsp vanilla

Instructions
- In a medium sized saucepan, at medium heat, bring the oats and water to the boil.
- Turn down the heat and simmer for five to ten minutes, until the water is absorbed.
- Take the saucepan off the heat and add the cinnamon, vanilla and coconut milk.
- Simmer again for two to three minutes, whilst stirring and thoroughly mixing to a smooth creamy consistency.
- Pour into bowls immediately and top with your favourite fruit and/or other toppings

## Lunch

### Arugula Salad

Ingredients

Salad:

- 5 oz. baby arugula (full grown works too)

- 2/3 cup sliced almonds, toasted
- 1/2 cup dried cranberries (sweetened variety)
- 1/2 cup shaved parmesan (1.5 oz)

Dressing:
- 1/4 cup extra virgin olive oil
- 2 Tbsp fresh lemon juice or 2.5 Tbsp balsamic vinegar
- 1 Tbsp honey
- Salt and freshly ground black pepper, to taste

Instructions
- Make the dressing: In a small mixing bowl whisk together olive oil, lemon juice, honey and season with salt and pepper to taste.
- Chill dressing for 15 minutes if time allows.
- To assemble salad: Toss the arugula with about 2/3 of the dressing then on a serving platter or individual salad plates layer half the arugula, half the almonds, half the cranberries and half the parmesan.
- Repeat layering then drizzle with remaining 1/3 of the dressing. Serve right away.

# Dinner

Pinto Beans

Preparation Time: 15 Minutes
Cooking Time: 1hour 30 Minutes
Soaking Time: 8 Hours
Serves: 8-12
Ingredients
- 2 cups dry pinto beans
- 1 tablespoon avocado oil
- ½ white onion, chopped
- 1½ teaspoons cumin
- 8 cups water, more as needed
- ½ teaspoon oregano
- 2 teaspoons fine sea salt, more to taste

- Freshly ground black pepper
- 1 tablespoon lime juice, more to taste

Instructions

- Place the beans in a large colander and sort through them to remove and discard any stones or debris. Rinse them well and transfer them to a large bowl. Cover with 2 to 3 inches of water and discard any beans that float. Soak at room temperature for 8 hours or overnight. Drain and rinse.
- In a large pot or Dutch oven, heat the oil over medium heat. Add the onion and sauté until soft, about 5 minutes. If you like spicy beans, add the jalapeño with the onion.
- Stir in the cumin and then add the beans, water, oregano, salt, and several grinds of pepper and bring to a boil. Reduce the heat and simmer, uncovered, until the beans are tender. The timing will depend on the freshness of your beans. I like to check mine starting at 1 hour and every 15 minutes after that. Add more liquid to the pot, as needed, to keep the beans submerged. I like to cook my pinto beans until they're starting to fall apart and the bean liquid around them has thickened.
- Turn off the heat and stir in the lime juice. Season the beans to taste with more salt (I typically add ½ to 1 additional teaspoon), more pepper, and chili powder, if desired. Garnish with cilantro, if using. Store the beans in an airtight container in the fridge for up to 5 days, or freeze them for up to 3 months.

# Day 4

## Breakfast

Potato Salad

Preparation Time: 20 Minutes
Cooking Time: 20 Minutes
Ingredients
- 800g small new potato
- 3 shallots, finely chopped
- 1 tbsp small capers (optional)
- 2 tbsp cornichons, finely chopped (optional)
- 3 tbsp mayonnaise, or to taste
- 3 tbsp extra-virgin olive oil
- 1 tbsp white wine vinegar
- small handful parsley leaves, roughly chopped

Instructions
- Boil the potatoes in salted water for 20 mins until just cooked, drain, then cool.
- Cut the potatoes into chunks, then throw into a bowl with the shallots, capers and cornichons, if using. Add enough mayonnaise to bind, then mix together the olive oil and vinegar and add just enough to give a little sharpness to the salad. Stir in the finely chopped parsley and serve.

## Lunch

Veggie Tots

Preparation Time: 15 Minutes
Cooking Time: 30 Minutes
Total Time: 45 Minutes
Servings: 6
Ingredients
- 1 cup chopped broccoli , save the stems for baked sticks/rounds

- 1 cup chopped cauliflower , save the stems for baked sticks/rounds
- ½ cup potato , about 1 medium peeled potato
- ½ cup white beans
- ½ cup breadcrumbs
- 1 teaspoon minced onion , either red or yellow/white works
- ¾ teaspoon sea salt
- ¼ teaspoon ground black pepper
- Creamy Chive Dip (optional but recommended):
- 1 ½ cups cashews
- 1 cup water
- 2 tablespoons lemon juice
- 1 tablespoon white distilled vinegar
- 1 clove garlic
- 1 teaspoon sea salt
- ½ cup chopped chives

Instructions
- Preheat the oven to 400 F/ 205 C
- Boil potato for about 6-8 minutes, until just able to put fork in it. Blanch broccoli and cauliflower by dropping them in the boiling water for about a minute. You could also cook the potato in the microwave, and blanch the broccoli and cauliflower. Or cook them all in the microwave. See notes for instructions on using frozen veggies.
- While this is cooking, you can use the stems of the broccoli and cauliflower by cutting them into sticks or rounds. Mix with a drizzle of olive oil, dash of sea salt and black pepper. Put on a parchment lined cookie sheet and set aside.
- Strain the potato, broccoli and cauliflower and put in a food processor with the other ingredients.
- Pulse until mixture is crumbly and sticks together.
- Form into tot shapes. I used about a heaping tablespoon for each.
- Bake on a parchment lined cookie sheet for 30-35 minutes, or until the edges are browning. Also put the cookie sheet

with the stems in the oven at the same time. Bake these for about 20 minutes, or until you get the texture you like.
- While baking, if making the dip, put all ingredients except the chives into a blender and blending until nice and smooth. Add in the chives and pulse to incorporate.
- When the tots and stems are done. Serve with the dip!

## Dinner

### Caprese Salad

Prep Time: 5 Minutes
Cooking Time: 29 Minutes
Total Time: 25 Minutes
Servings: 8
Ingredients
- 2 c balsamic vinegar
- 3 whole ripe tomatoes, sliced thick
- 12 oz. mozzarella cheese, sliced thick
- Fresh basil leaves
- Olive oil, for drizzling
- Kosher salt and freshly ground black pepper

Instructions
- Bring the balsamic vinegar to a boil over medium-low heat in a small saucepan. Cook for 10 to 20 minutes, or until the balsamic has reduced to a thicker glaze. Remove it from the heat and transfer to a bowl or cruet. Allow to cool.
- 2When you're ready to serve, arrange tomato and mozzarella slices on a platter. Arrange basil leaves between the slices. Drizzle olive oil over the top of the salad, getting a little bit on each slice. Do the same with the balsamic reduction, making designs if you want. Store extra balsamic reduction in fridge for a later use.
- 3End with a sprinkling of kosher salt and black pepper. Serve as a lunch, with crusty bread, or serve alongside a beef main course for dinner.

# Day 5

## breakfast

Cobb Salad

Preparation Time: 20 Minutes
Total Time: 20 Minutes
Servings: 4
Ingredients
- 6 slices bacon
- 1/2 head romaine
- 1/2 head Boston lettuce
- 1 small bunch frisée (curly endive)
- 1/2 bunch watercress, coarse stems discarded
- 2 ripe avocados, seed removed, peeled, and cut into 1/2-inch pieces
- 1 whole skinless boneless chicken breast (about 3/4 pound total), halved, cooked, and diced (see How to Poach Chicken)
- 1 tomato, seeded and chopped fine
- 2 hard-boiled large eggs, separated, the yolk finely chopped and the white finely chopped (see How to Make Hard Boiled Eggs)
- 2 tablespoons chopped fresh chives
- 1/3 cup red wine vinegar
- 1 tablespoon Dijon-style mustard
- 1 to 2 teaspoons sugar
- Salt and pepper
- 2/3 cup extra virgin olive oil
- 1/2 cup finely grated Roquefort cheese

Instructions
- in a skillet on medium heat until crisp on both sides. Remove from skillet and lay out on paper towels to absorb the excess fat. Allow the bacon to cool. Crumble the bacon and set aside.

- In a large salad bowl, toss together well the various lettuces and watercress.
- Arrange the chicken, the bacon, the tomato, and the avocado decoratively over the greens and garnish the salad with the chopped egg and the chives.
- In a small bowl whisk together the vinegar, the mustard, and salt and pepper to taste, add the oil in a slow stream, whisking, and whisk the dressing until it is emulsified. Stir in the Roquefort. Add sugar to taste, 1/2 teaspoon at a time. Whisk the dressing. Serve separately or toss in with the salad.

# Lunch

## Salmon Milano With Pesto Butter

Preparation Time: 5 Minutes
Cooking Time: 15 Minutes
Total Time: 20 Minutes
Servings: 4
Ingredients
- 1 lb salmon
- 2 tablespoon butter
- 1 tablespoon pesto
- .1 oz dill weed
- Instructions
- Preheat your oven or air fryer to 400 degrees. For copycat dish, mash together the butter and pesto in a small bowl with a fork.
- Copycat: Place salmon skin side down on a baking pan, and spread the pesto-butter mixture on top, then add fresh dill.
- Costco take and bake: remove lid.
- Bake for 12-16 minutes in oven, or 5-10 minutes in air fryer, depending on thickness. Enjoy!

# Dinner

## Pineapple Yoghurt

Cooking Time: 5 Min
Servings: 12
Ingredients
- 3 cups plain Greek yogurt
- 1 3.4 oz box instant vanilla pudding mix dry mix only
- 20 oz can crushed pineapple in juice, undrained

Instructions
- Combine yogurt and dry vanilla pudding mix together in a large bowl.
- Stir until all traces of pudding mix have disappeared.
- Stir in the pineapple, including the juice, until well combined.
- Cover and refrigerate for 3 hours.

# Day 6

## Breakfast

### Potato Chips

Preparation Time: 40 Minutes
Cooking Time: 20 Minutes
Total Time: 1hr
Servings: 8
Ingredients
- 4 medium potatoes, peeled and sliced paper-thin
- 3 tablespoons salt, plus more to taste
- 1 quart oil for deep frying

Instructions
- Transfer potato slices to a large bowl of cold water as you slice them.
- Drain slices and rinse under cold water. Refill the bowl with water, add 3 tablespoons salt, and put slices back in the bowl. Let potatoes soak in the salty water for at least 30 minutes.
- Drain and rinse slices again. Pat dry.
- Heat oil in a deep-fryer to 365 degrees F (185 degrees C).
- Working in small batches, fry potato slices until golden. Remove with a slotted spoon and drain on paper towels. Continue until all of the slices are fried.
- Season potato chips with additional salt if desired.

## Lunch

### Bruleed Orange

Preparation Time: 5 Minutes
Cooking Time: 10 Minutes
Total Time: 15 Minutes
Servings: 2
Ingredients

- 2 oranges cut in half
- ½ cup sugar

Instructions
- Cut each orange in half. Use a sharp knife to cut around the orange's insides to separate them from the rind. Cut diagonally along the internal lines that separate the orange slices to loosen them. Let any excess orange juice drip off.
- Place the orange face down in a bowl of sugar to make a thick sugar coating on the top of the fruit. Use the brûlée torch to caramelize the sugar, but not burn it. Keep the torch about a half inch away from the sugar and move in a continuous circular motion.
- Let the topping cool for a minute before cracking into it with a spoon. Serve right away and enjoy!

# Dinner

## Nacho Pizza

Preparation Time: 20 Minutes
Cooking Time: 15 Minutes
Total Time: 35 Minutes
Servings: 4
Ingredients
- 1 pound lean ground beef
- 1 (1.25 ounce) package taco seasoning mix
- 1 (12 inch) parbaked thin pizza crust
- 5 tablespoons queso dip
- 1 cup shredded aged Cheddar cheese
- 1 jalapeno pepper, seeded and minced
- 4 green onions, diced
- 4 tablespoons salsa
- ½ cup crushed tortilla chips
- 2 tablespoons sour cream, or to taste

Instructions
- Preheat the oven to 450 degrees F (230 degrees C).

- cook beef in a large skillet under no longer pink, about 5 minutes. Drain. Stir in seasoning mix until evenly combined.
- Place pizza crust on a work surface. Spread ⬚ueso dip evenly over the crust. Top with Cheddar cheese, cooked beef mixture, jalapeno, and green onions. Spoon salsa onto the pizza in random spots, making sure it's not mixed in with the other toppings. Sprinkle crushed tortilla chips on top.
- Bake in the preheated oven directly on the middle oven rack until cheese is hot and melted, about 8 minutes. Serve with sour cream.

# Day 7

## Breakfast

Lobster Salad

Preparation Time: 9 Minutes
Cooking Time: 1 Minute
Total Time: 10 Minutes
Serving 4
Ingredients
- 1 1/2 pounds cooked lobster meat approximately 3 1/2 cups, cut into 3/4 inch pieces
- 1/3 cup mayonnaise
- 1 1/2 tablespoons lemon juice
- 1/4 cup celery finely chopped, use the tender inner stalks
- 1 tablespoon chives thinly sliced, plus more for garnish
- salt and pepper to taste

Instructions
- Place the lobster meat, mayonnaise, lemon juice, celery, chives, salt and pepper in a bowl. Stir gently to combine.
- Serve immediately, or chill for up to 4 hours. Garnish with additional chives before serving.

## Lunch

Watermelon Ice

Preparation Time: 6 Hours
Total Time: 6 Hours
Servings: 6
Ingredients
- 1kg (around ½ watermelon) watermelon flesh (chopped)
- Juice of 1 lime
- Lime zest
- (I used the zest of half a lime because we like the taste of lime but you may not want to add as much)

## Instructions

- Place the watermelon, lime juice and zest into a food processor /blender and blend until smooth.
- Transfer the mixture to a shallow, freezable container and place in freezer.
- After two hours, gently scrape the top layer with a spoon. Once you get to the unfrozen mixture pop it back in the freezer. Repeat after another 2 hours.
- Freeze until solid (around 6 hours depending on surface area of container)
- Scrape with a spoon and serve

# Dinner

Chocolate Bread

Preparation Time: 20 Minutes
Cooking Time: 1 Hr
Total Time: 1hr 20 Minutes
Serving : 1
Ingredients

- ½ cup dutch process cocoa
- 1 ¾ cups all purpose flour
- 6 tablespoons dark brown sugar
- 6 tablespoons granulated sugar
- 1 ½ teaspoons baking powder
- ¾ teaspoon baking soda
- ¼ teaspoon salt
- 1 cup buttermilk
- 2 large eggs room temperature
- ½ cup vegetable oil
- 1 teaspoon vanilla extract
- ¾ cup semi sweet chocolate chips divided

## Instructions

- Preheat the oven to 350 degrees Fahrenheit. Spray a 9×5 bread pan with cooking spray and set aside.

- In a large bowl, whisk together the cocoa, flour, both sugars, baking powder, baking soda, and salt.
- Add the buttermilk, eggs, oil, and vanilla. Mix until combined. Fold in ½ cup of the chocolate chips.
- Pour the batter into the prepared pan and top with the remaining ¼ cup of chocolate chips.
- Bake for 55-60 minutes, until a toothpick comes out clean from the center.
- Let cool completely before slicing.

# Day 8

## Breakfast

### Oatmeal Butterscotch Bars

Cooking Time: 40 Minutes
Ingredients
- 1cup flour
- 1teaspoon baking soda
- 1/2teaspoon salt
- 3/4teaspoon cinnamon
- 1cup butter, softened (plus a little more to grease the pan)
- 3/4cup white sugar
- 2eggs
- 1teaspoon vanilla (or a bit more)
- 3cups regular oatmeal, uncooked
- 1(12 ounce) package butterscotch chips

Instructions
- Preheat oven to 350°F.
- Grease a 9x13 pan with butter.
- Combine flour, soda, salt and cinnamon.
- In a large mixing bowl cream butter, then add sugar and mix until fluffy.
- Add eggs and vanilla and beat well.
- Gradually add flour mixture.
- Stir in oatmeal and the butterscotch chips.
- Spread in prepared pan and bake for 22 to 28 minutes.
- If they seem to be getting to brown on the edges, and are still ?uite gooey in the center lower the oven temp to 325°F for the last 10 minutes or so.

## Lunch

### Pizza Sticks

Preparation Time: 5 Minutes
Baking Time: 12 Minutes
Total Time: 17 Minutes
Ingredients

- 1 (12-oz.) refrigerated thin pizza crust
- 1 (10.5-oz.) container tomato bruschetta topping
- 1 cup (4 oz.) shredded Italian cheese blend

Instructions

- Top 1 (12-oz.) refrigerated thin pizza crust with 1 (5-oz.) container tomato bruschetta topping. Sprinkle evenly with 1 cup (4 oz.) shredded Italian cheese blend. Bake at 450°, directly on oven rack, 12 minutes or until crust is golden and cheese is bubbly. Cut pizza in half, and cut each half lengthwise into 2-inch strips.
- Note: For testing purposes only, we used Buitoni Classic Bruschetta.

## Dinner

### Cioppino

Servings: 4-6
Prep Time: 45 Minutes
Cook Time: 1 Hour
Total Time: 1 Hour 45 Minutes
Ingredients

- ¼ cup + 2 tablespoons extra-virgin olive oil, divided
- ⅔ cup finely chopped shallots, from about 3 shallots
- 3 cloves garlic, minced
- 1 cup white wine
- 1 (28 oz) can crushed tomatoes
- 2 (8 oz) bottles clam juice
- 2 teaspoons sugar
- 1¾ teaspoons salt, divided
- ½ teaspoon crushed red pepper flakes
- ½ teaspoon dried oregano
- 7 sprigs fresh thyme, plus 1 teaspoon fresh chopped thyme

- 1½ pounds firm-fleshed fish fillets, such as halibut, cod, salmon, snapper, etc., cut into 2-inch pieces
- 3 tablespoons unsalted butter
- 1½ pounds (about 18) littleneck clams, scrubbed (see note)
- 1½ pounds extra large raw shrimp, peeled and deveined
- Fresh chopped Italian parsley, for garnish (optional)

Instructions

- Preheat the oven to 400°F and set an oven rack in the middle position. Line a baking sheet with aluminum foil and set aside.
- In a large pot, heat ¼ cup of the oil over medium heat. Add the shallots and cook, stirring frequently, until soft and translucent, about 5 minutes. Add the garlic and cook, stirring constantly, for 1 minute more. Do not brown.
- Add the wine and increase the heat to high. Boil until the wine is reduced by about half, 3 to 4 minutes.
- Add the crushed tomatoes, clam juice, sugar, 1 teaspoon of the salt, red pepper flakes, oregano, thyme sprigs, and 1 cup of water. Bring to a boil; reduce the heat and simmer, covered, for 25 minutes.
- Meanwhile, while the stew is simmering, toss the fish with the remaining 2 tablespoons oil and remaining ¾ teaspoon salt. Arrange the fish on the prepared baking sheet and bake for about 10 minutes, or until just cooked through. Cover and keep warm until ready to serve.
- When the stew is done simmering, remove and discard the thyme sprigs and stir in the butter. Add the clams and bring the stew back to a simmer. Cover and cook for about 6 minutes, until the clams have mostly opened. Gently stir in the shrimp and bring the stew back to a simmer; cover and cook until the shrimp are just cooked through and the clams are completely opened, about 5 minutes. Discard any unopened clams. Add the chopped thyme, then taste the stew and adjust seasoning, if necessary.
- Divide the warm fish into serving bowls. Ladle the stew over top, dividing the clams and shrimp evenly amongst

the bowls. Garnish with parsley, if using, and serve with garlic bread, focaccia, or a baguette for sopping up the broth. Set out a second bowl for shells and plenty of napkins.

- Make Ahead: The stew, without seafood, can be made 2 days ahead and stored in the refrigerator, covered. When ready to serve, bake the fish and bring the stew to a simmer before adding the seafood.

# Day 9

## Breakfast

Vegetable Beef Soup

Cooking Time: 1hr 10 Minutes
Preparation Time: 20 Minutes
Total Time: 1hr 30 Minutes
Servings: 8
Ingredients
- 1 1/2 lbs beef stew meat
- 2 1/2 Tbsp olive oil, divided
- Salt and freshly ground black pepper
- 1 3/4 cups chopped yellow onion (1 large)
- 1 1/4 cups peeled and chopped carrots (3 medium)
- 1 cup chopped celery (3 medium)
- 1 1/2 Tbsp minced garlic (4 cloves)
- 8 cups low-sodium beef broth or chicken broth
- 2 (14 oz.) cans diced tomatoes
- 1 1/2 tsp dried basil
- 1 tsp dried oregano
- 1/2 tsp dried thyme
- 1 lb red or yellow potatoes, chopped into 3/4-inch cubes
- 1 1/2 cups (5 oz.) chopped green beans (trim ends first)
- 1 1/2 cups frozen corn
- 1 cup frozen peas
- 1/3 cup chopped fresh parsley

Instructions
- Heat 1 Tbsp olive oil in a large pot over medium-high heat.
- Dab beef dry with paper towels, season with salt and pepper then add half of the beef to pot and brown about 4 minutes, turning halfway through.
- Transfer to a plate add another 1/2 Tbsp oil to pot and repeat process with remaining half of beef.

- Add another 1 Tbsp oil to now empty pot then add onions, carrots, and celery then saute 3 minutes, add garlic saute 1 minute longer.
- Pour in broth, tomatoes, browned beef, basil, oregano, thyme and season with salt and pepper. Bring to a boil then reduce heat to low, cover and simmer, stirring once or twice throughout, for 30 minutes.
- Add potatoes then continue to simmer, covered, 20 minutes (you can also add green beans with potatoes if you like them very soft).
- Stir in green beans and simmer 15 minutes longer, or until all of the veggies and beef are tender.
- Pour in corn and peas and simmer until heated through, about 5 minutes. Stir in parsley and serve warm.
- Recipe source: Cooking Classy

# Lunch

## Pumpkin Soup

Preparation Time: 20 Mins
Cooking Time: 25 Minutes
Servings: 6
Ingredients
- 2 tablespoon olive oil
- 2 onions, finely chopped
- 1kg pumpkin or squash (try kabocha), peeled, deseeded and chopped into chunks
- 700ml vegetable stock or chicken stock
- 150ml double cream

## For the croutons

- 2 tablespoon olive oil
- 4 slices wholemeal seeded bread, crusts removed
- handful pumpkin seeds

instructions

- Heat 2 tbsp olive oil in a large saucepan, then gently cook 2 finely chopped onions for 5 mins, until soft but not coloured.
- Add 1kg pumpkin or squash, cut into chunks, to the pan, then carry on cooking for 8-10 mins, stirring occasionally until it starts to soften and turn golden.
- Pour 700ml vegetable or chicken stock into the pan and season with salt and pepper. Bring to the boil, then simmer for 10 mins until the squash is very soft.
- Pour 150ml double cream into the pan, bring back to the boil, then purée with a hand blender. For an extra-velvety consistency you can pour the soup through a fine sieve. The soup can now be frozen for up to 2 months.
- To make the croutons: cut 4 slices wholemeal seeded bread into small squares.
- Heat 2 tbsp olive oil in a frying pan, then fry the bread until it starts to become crisp.
- Add a handful of pumpkin seeds to the pan, then cook for a few mins more until they are toasted. These can be made a day ahead and stored in an airtight container.
- Reheat the soup if needed, taste for seasoning, then serve scattered with croutons and seeds and drizzled with more olive oil, if you want.

# Dinner

## Layered Salad

Preparation Time: 30 Minutes
Servings: 12
Total Time: 30 Minutes
Ingredients

For the salad

- 2 head iceberg lettuce, chopped
- 8 oz. fluid baby spinach, washed and dried

- Salt and pepper, to taste
- 8 whole hard boiled eggs, chopped
- 16 oz. bacon, cooked and chopped
- 4 whole tomatoes, chopped
- 1 bunch green onions, thinly sliced
- 8 oz. cheddar cheese, grated
- 10 oz. frozen peas, partially thawed

## For dressing

- ½ c. mayonnaise
- ½ c. sour cream
- 1 tablespoon. Sugar
- Chopped fresh dill, for topping

## Instructions

- To make the salad: Layer the salad ingredients in a clear glass bowl starting with the lettuce, concentrating the ingredients around the perimeter of the bowl and filling in the center with lettuce, if needed. End with the layer of peas.
- To make the dressing: Combine ingredients in a separate bowl and mix well. Pour over the top of the peas and spread to cover, bringing the dressing all the way out to the edges of the bowl. Sprinkle with fresh dill.
- Cover and refrigerate for up to 8 hours. Toss just before serving.

# Day 10

## Breakfast

Glazed Lemon Loaf

Preparation Time: 15 Minutes
Cooking Time: 1hr 5 Minutes
Cooling: 3 Hrs
Total: 4 Hrs 20 Minutes
Servings: 8
Ingredients
Dry ingredients

- 2 cups plain flour / all-purpose flour
- 4 tsp baking powder
- 1/8 tsp salt
- Wet ingredients
- 1 cup plain yogurt
- 2 large eggs
- 75g / 5 tbsp unsalted butter
- 1/4 cup vegetable or canola oil
- 2 tbsp lemon zest
- 1/4 cup lemon juice
- 1 1/4 cups caster sugar / superfine sugar
- 1/2 tsp vanilla extract
- 1 1/2 tsp lemon extract
- Glaze (optional)
- 1 cup soft icing sugar/powdered sugar
- 3 – 3 1/2 tsp+ lemon juice

Instructions

- Preheat oven to 180°C/350°F (160°C fan-forced). Grease then line a 21 x 11 x 7 cm (8.5 x 4.5 x 2.75") with baking / parchment paper. (Note 4)
- Batter – Whisk Dry ingredients in a large bowl. Whisk Wet ingredients in a separate bowl. Pour Wet ingredients into

the Dry ingredients. Whisk just until lump free. Pour into the prepared loaf pan then smooth the surface.

- Bake 45 minutes uncovered. Loosely cover with foil then bake a further 20 minutes or until a skewer inserted comes out clean.
- Cool & glaze – Stand 10 min in pan then turn out onto a cooling rack. Fully cool before glazing (~3 hours). Use a spoon to spread and coax lovely glaze drips down the side! Cut thick slices and serve.
- Glaze – Whisk ingredients until combined and smooth, a thick smooth frosting that will drip thickly, not be transparent. Start with 3 1/2 teaspoons lemon juice, and add 1/2 tsp extra, as needed. (Note 5 on thickness)

# Lunch

## Vanilla Smoothie

### Ingredients
- 2 frozen bananas , (peels removed before freezing)
- 2 scoops vanilla protein powder
- 1 cup vanilla almond milk
- 2 tablespoon real maple syrup
- ¼ cup walnuts
- 2 tablespoon flax seeds, ground or whole

### Instructions
- Blend up all ingredients in a food processor or blender.
- Use one of these insulated cold cups to keep your smoothie perfectly cold while drinking.
- Keeps in fridge for 2-3 days.

# Dinner

## Cinnamon rolls

Preparation time: 2 hours
Cooking time: 20 mins

Total time: 2 hours 20 mins
Servings: 9
Ingredients

For the dough:

- ¾ cup warm milk (whole milk or 2% preferred) (110 degrees F)
- 2 ¼ teaspoons quick rise or active yeast (1/4-ounce package yeast)
- ¼ cup granulated sugar
- 1 egg plus 1 egg yolk, at room temperature
- ¼ cup butter, melted (I prefer salted, but unsalted works, too)
- 3 cups bread flour, plus more for dusting
- 3/4 teaspoon salt

For the filling:

- 2/3 cup dark brown sugar (light brown sugar also works)
- 1 ½ tablespoons ground cinnamon
- ¼ cup butter, softened
- For the cream cheese frosting:
- 4 oz cream cheese, softened
- 3 tablespoons butter, softened
- ¾ cup powdered sugar
- ½ teaspoon vanilla extract

Instructions
- Warm milk to around 110 degrees F. I like to do this by placing milk in a microwave safe bowl and microwaving it for 40-45 seconds. It should be like warm bath water. Transfer warm milk to the bowl of an electric mixer and sprinkle yeast on top. Add in sugar, egg, egg yolk and melted butter. Mix until well combined. Next stir in flour and salt with a wooden spoon until a dough begins to form.

- Place dough hook on stand mixer and knead dough on medium speed for 8 minutes. Dough should form into a nice ball and be slightly sticky. If it's TOO sticky (meaning it's sticking to the bottom of the mixer, add in 2 tablespoons more bread flour.) If you don't want to use an electric mixer, you can use your hands to knead the dough for 8-10 minutes on a well-floured surface.
- Transfer dough ball to a well-oiled bowl, cover with plastic wrap and a warm towel. Allow dough to rise for 1 hour to 1 ½ hours, or until doubled in size. This may more or less time depending the humidity and temperature in your home.
- After dough has doubled in size, transfer dough to a well-floured surface and roll out into a 14x9 inch rectangle. Spread softened butter over dough, leaving a ¼ inch margin at the far side of the dough.
- In a small bowl, mix together brown sugar and cinnamon. Use your hands to sprinkle mixture over the buttered dough, then rub the brown sugar mixture into the butter.
- Tightly roll dough up, starting from the 9-inch side and place seam side down making sure to seal the edges of the dough as best you can. You will probably need to cut off about an inch off the ends of the dough as the ends won't be as full of cinnamon sugar as we'd want it to be.
- Cut into 1 inch sections with a serrated knife or floss. You should get 9 large pieces.
- Place cinnamon rolls in a greased 9x9 inch baking pan or round 9 inch cake pan. (I also recommend lining the pan with parchment paper as well, in case any of the filling ends up leaking out.) Cover with plastic wrap and a warm towel and let rise again for 30-45 minutes.
- Preheat oven to 350 degrees F. Remove plastic wrap and towel and bake cinnamon rolls for 20-25 minutes or until just slightly golden brown on the edges. You want to underbake them a little so they stay soft in the middle, that's why we want them just slightly golden brown. Allow

them to cool for 5-10 minutes before frosting. Makes 9 cinnamon rolls.

- To make the frosting: In the bowl of an electric mixer, combine cream cheese, butter, powdered sugar and vanilla extract. Beat until smooth and fluffy. Spread over cinnamon rolls and serve immediately. Enjoy!

# Day 11

## Breakfast

Roasted Green Beans

Preparation Time: 5 Minutes
Cooking Time: 15 Minutes
Total Time: 20 Minutes
Servings: 4
Ingredients
- 1 pound (16 ounces) green beans or haricots verts
- 2 teaspoons extra-virgin olive oil
- Scant ¼ teaspoon fine sea salt
- Instructions
- Preheat the oven to 425 degrees Fahrenheit and line a large, rimmed baking sheet with parchment paper for easy cleanup.
- Wash and trim the rough ends off the green beans. Pat them very dry with clean tea towels (wet green beans turn soggy in the oven).
- Place the prepared green beans on your baking sheet. Drizzle the olive oil over the beans and sprinkle the salt all over. Use your hands to toss until all of the beans are lightly coated in oil. Arrange the green beans across the pan in a single layer.
- Roast for 14 to 16 minutes, undisturbed, until they are crisp-tender with some golden, caramelized spots. (If using slender haricots verts, they may be ready a couple of minutes earlier.)
- Transfer to a serving dish and enjoy with any desired accompaniments (see recipe notes for seasoning suggestions). Roasted green beans are best enjoyed while warm, but will keep in the refrigerator, covered, for 4 to 5 days.

# Lunch

## Glazed Orange Carrots

Preparation Time: 5 Mins
Cooking Time: 10 Mins
Ingredients
- 600g baby carrot
- 1 ½ tbsp butter
- 3 tbsp orange juice
- handful parsley leaves, chopped

Instructions
- Trim the carrots and cook in boiling water for 4-6 mins until just tender, then drain. Melt the butter in a large frying pan, add the drained carrots, then fry over a high heat for 1 min. Pour over the orange juice and cook for a further 2-3 mins, bubbling the sauce and stirring to thoroughly coat the carrots. Finally, stir in the chopped parsley and serve.

# Dinner

## Broccoli Salad

Preparation Time: 15 Minutes
Cook Time: 10 Minutes
Total Time: 25 Minutes
Servings: 8
Ingredients
- ½ pound bacon
- 2 heads fresh broccoli, cut into bite-sized pieces
- 1 small red onion, sliced into bite-sized pieces
- ¾ cup raisins
- ¾ cup sliced almonds
- 1 cup mayonnaise
- ½ cup white sugar
- 2 tablespoons white wine vinegar

# Instructions

- Gather all ingredients.
- Place bacon in a deep skillet and cook over medium-high heat until evenly brown, 7 to 10 minutes; drain, cool, and crumble.
- Combine bacon, broccoli, onion, raisins, and almonds together in a bowl; mix well.
- To prepare the dressing: Mix mayonnaise, sugar, and vinegar together until smooth.
- Stir into the salad
- Let chill before serving, if desired.

# Day 12

## Breakfast

### Creamy Corn Pudding

Preparation Time: 10 Minutes
Cook Time: 1 Hr
Servings: 8
Ingredients
- 5 eggs
- 1/3 cup butter(melted)
- ¼ cup white sugar
- ½ cup milk
- 4 tablespoons cornstarch
- 1(15.25 oz) can whole kernel corn
- 2(14.75 oz) cans cream-style corn

Instructions
- Preheat oven to 400 Degrees Fahrenheit. Grease a 2-Quart casserole dish.
- In a large bowl, lightly beat eggs. Add sugar, milk, and melted butter. Add the cornstarch and whisk until fully incorporated. Add corn and creamed corn. Mix well. Pour mixture into the prepared casserole dish.
- Bake in the oven for one hour at 400 degrees F.
- Enjoy!

## Lunch

### Bagel

Preparation Time: 30 Mins
Cook Time: 35 Mins
Servings: 10
- Put the dough in a lightly oiled bowl and cover with a piece of oiled cling film. Place in a warm area and leave until

doubled in size, about 1 hr, then uncover and tip onto your work surface.

## Ingredients

- 7g sachet fast-action dried yeast
- 500g strong white flour, plus a little extra for shaping
- 2 tbsp light brown soft sugar
- a little oil, for greasing
- 1 tbsp bicarbonate of soda
- 1 egg white, to glaze
- seeds of your choice for the topping

## Instructions

- Mix the yeast with 300ml lukewarm water. Put the flour, sugar and 1 tsp salt in a large bowl and mix together. Pour over the yeasty liquid and mix into a rough dough.
- Tip out onto the work surface and knead together until smooth and elastic – this should take around 10 mins.
- Put the dough in a lightly oiled bowl and cover with a piece of oiled cling film. Place in a warm area and leave until doubled in size, about 1 hr, then uncover and tip onto your work surface.
- Divide the dough into 10 portions and form into balls – I like to weigh them to make sure that they're all the same size. Line up on two parchment-lined baking trays and cover lightly with cling film.
- Leave for around 30 mins or until risen and puffy, then remove the cling film.
- Use a floured finger to make a hole in the centre of each bagel, swirling it around to stretch the dough a little, but being careful not to knock out too much air. Heat oven to 180C/160C fan/gas 4.
- Fill a large saucepan with water and bring to the boil. Add the bicarbonate of soda to alkalise the water (see tip, below). Place 1-2 of the bagels in the water at a time and boil for 1 min (2 mins if you want a chewier bagel), turning

over halfway through. Using a slotted spoon, lift out the bagels, drain well and place back on the baking tray.

- Brush the bagels with the egg white and sprinkle with your chosen seeds. Bake for 20-25 mins or until golden brown. Transfer to a wire rack to cool before eating. They will keep for 3-4 days, or freeze for two months

# Dinner

## Fish Nuggets

Preparation Time: 10 Mins
Cook Time: 10 Mins
Total Time
20 Mins
Ingredients

- 500 g Fish Cod, cut into bite-sized chunks
- 100 g Plain Flour
- 1 tsp Garlic Powder
- 1 tsp Paprika
- 1 tsp Dried Thyme
- 1 tsp Salt
- 1 tsp Black Pepper
- 2 large Eggs Beaten
- 150 g Breadcrumbs
- Vegetable Oil For frying

Instructions

- In a mixing bowl, combine flour, garlic powder, paprika, thyme, salt, and pepper.
- Beat eggs in a separate bowl.
- Put breadcrumbs in a third bowl.
- Coat each piece of fish with the flour mixture, then dip in beaten eggs, and coat with breadcrumbs, pressing lightly to help the coating adhere.
- Heat a large frying pan over medium-high heat and add enough oil to cover the base.

- Once the oil is hot, fry the fish nuggets in batches for 2-3 minutes on each side until they turn golden brown and crispy.
- Use a slotted spoon to transfer the cooked fish nuggets to a plate lined with paper towels to remove excess oil.
- Serve hot with tartar sauce or your preferred dipping sauce.

# Day 13

## Breakfast

### Lobster Tail

Preparation Time: 10 Mins
Cook Time: 10 Mins
Total Time: 20 Mins
Servings: 4
Instructions
- 4 lobster tails
- salt and pepper
- 1/4 cup butter melted
- 3 garlic cloves minced
- 1/2 teaspoon paprika
- 1 teaspoon thyme minced
- 1 teaspoon rosemary minced
- 1 teaspoon parsley chopped

Instructions
- Preheat the oven to broil or 500 degrees. Start by preparing the lobster. Using kitchen shears butterfly the tail by cutting down the center. Loosen the meat and pull the lobster meat upward. Salt and pepper the meat and set on a baking sheet.
- In a small bowl whisk together the melted butter, garlic, paprika, thyme, rosemary, and parsley. Spread evenly on each lobster tail.
- Broil the lobster tails for about 8-10 minutes or until the meat is opaque and lightly brown on the top. Serve with melted butter if desired.

## Lunch

### Parmesan Garlic Crumbed Fish

Preparation Time: 5 Mins

Cook Time: 7 Mins
Total Time: 12 Mins
Ingredients

- 2 firm white fish fillets
- 2 tbsp dijon mustard
- Olive oil spray
- Salt and pepper
- Crump
- 1/2 cup panko breadcrumbs
- 1 tbsp parsley
- 1/3 cup (30g) parmesan, finely grated
- 1 garlic clove , minced
- 1 tbsp olive oil
- Pinch of salt

Instructions

- Preheat grill / broiler on high.
- Combine the Crumb ingredients and mix well to combine.
- Sprinkle both sides of fish with salt and pepper, then spread the mustard on the top of each fillet (top only).
- Press the mustard smeared side of the fish into the crumb mixture. Press down firmly to make it stick. Then spray with oil (for extra golden crumb!).
- Drizzle 1/2 tbsp oil in a skillet and preheat on the stove over high heat.
- Once skillet is hot, place the fillets in the hot pan then place under the grill / broiler (about 5"/15cm from the heat source) for 5 - 6 minutes until the crumb is golden and the fish is cooked, rotating as re?uired. Fish should flake in centre once cooked.
- Oven option: bake at 220C/390F for 10 - 12 minutes, then finish under the grill/broiler on high to make the crumb golden.
- Serve immediately with lemon wedges!

# Dinner

## Meatballs

Preparation Time: 25 Minutes
Cook Time: 20mins
Total Time: 45 Minutes
Ingredients
- 1/2 cup plain breadcrumbs
- 1/2 cup grated Parmesan
- 1/2 tsp garlic powder
- 1/2 tsp onion powder
- 1/2 tsp Italian seasoning
- 1/4 tsp salt
- 1/4 tsp pepper
- 2 large eggs
- 1/4 cup whole milk
- 1 lb. bulk Italian sausage
- 1 lb. ground beef

Instructions
- In a small bowl, combine the breadcrumbs, Parmesan, garlic powder, onion powder, Italian seasoning, salt, and pepper. In a separate small bowl, lightly whisk the two eggs.
- Add the breadcrumb mixture, eggs, milk, Italian sausage, and ground beef to a large bowl. Use your hands to mix the ingredients together until evenly combined. Avoid over mixing the meat.
- Let the meatball mixture rest for five minutes to allow the breadcrumbs time to soften. Divide and shape the meat into about 32 meatballs, approximately 2 Tbsp in volume each.
- Oven cooking instructions
- Preheat the oven to 400°F. Line a baking sheet with parchment. Place the meatballs on the baking sheet about one inch apart from each other.

- Bake the meatballs for about 15 minutes, or until lightly browned.
- Transfer the meatballs to a pot of red sauce and simmer for five more minutes in the sauce. If not using a red sauce, add an additional 3-5 minutes to the bake time, or until the meatballs are cooked through.

## Stove top cooking instruction

- Add a tablespoon of cooking oil to a large skillet and heat over medium. Once hot, swirl the oil to coat the surface of the skillet. Add half of the meatballs to the skillet.
- Cook the meatballs, turning every couple of minutes, until browned on all sides and cooked through. Repeat with the second batch of meatballs.
- Transfer the cooked meatballs to a pot of red sauce and simmer for a few minutes more before serving.

## Freezing instructions

- You can freeze the meatballs either cooked or uncooked. I prefer freezing them already cooked so they can go straight from the freezer into a pot of red sauce and then just simmer until heated through. Cooked meatballs should be completely cooled before placing in a gallon-sized freezer bag and transferred to the freezer.
- To freeze uncooked meatballs, place the raw meatballs on a parchment-lined baking sheet and freeze on the baking sheet until solid (1-2 hours) before transferring to a gallon-sized freezer bag for longer storage. Thaw completely before cooking.

# Day 14

## Breakfast

### Seekh Kababs

Cook Time: 45 Minutes
Preparation Time: 15 Minutes
Total Cook Time: 1 Hr
Servings: 6
Ingredients

- Oven temp: 375 F- 205 C
- 2 cups keema (minced mutton/lamb/beef)
- For marination:
- 1 tbsp vinegar
- 2 tbsp fenugreek leaves, chopped
- 1/2 tbsp garlic paste
- 1/2 tbsp ginger paste
- 1 1/2 tbsp salt
- 1/4 tbsp black pepper, powdered
- 1/4 tbsp garam masala
- 2 tbsp coriander leaves, chopped
- 1 tbsp green chillies, finely chopped
- Skewers to make the kebabs
- Oil for brushing
- chaat masala
- lemon wedges

Instructions

For the marination:

- In a large bowl, mix lamb mince with few Tbsp of vinegar, fenugreek leaves.
- Then add garlic paste, ginger paste, salt and black pepper as per taste.
- Add chopped coriander leaves and green chillies.

- Refrigerate the meat mixture, covered, to marinate for at least 5 hours.

For the kebabs:

- About 25 minutes before serving, shape the meat mixture into long 'tubes' around the skewers (seekhs) and place on to a grill over a drip tray or into the pre-heated oven (also on a drip tray) and bake for 20-25 minutes.
- Brush them with oil and cook for another 2 minutes.
- Using oven mittens or a cloth, carefully push the kebab from one end, on to a serving dish.
- Garnish with the chaat masala, onions, lemons and serve along with green chutney.

# Lunch

Pepper Poppers

Preparation Time: 10 Mins
Cook Time: 12 Mins
Total Time: 22 Mins
Ingredients
- 3.5 ounces Bacon Cubes / Strips
- 8 Mini Sweet Peppers
- ½ cup Grated Cheddar Cheese (50 grams)
- 7 ounces Cream Cheese (200 grams)
- A pinch of Black Pepper

Instructions
- Preheat the oven to 400°F/200°C.
- Meanwhile: Fry the bacon pieces until cooked.
- Rinse the peppers and cut each of them in half. Make sure to leave the green parts on. Remove the seeds and membranes.
- Mix together cheddar cheese, cream cheese, black pepper and bacon.

- Fill the peppers with the mixture and bake for 10-13 minutes or until heated through and the peppers are soft.
- Best served right away!

# Dinner

## Potato

Preparation Time: 5 Mins
Cook Time: 40 Mins
Total Time: 45 Mins
Ingredients
- Sweet Potatoes

## Topping Ideas:

- butter, or vegan butter
- sea salt
- chives
- dollop of greek yogurt, or tzatziki
- a scoop of guacamole
- a drizzle of creamy avocado cilantro lime dressing
- any of these stuffing ideas!

## Instructions
- Preheat the oven to 425°F and place a piece of foil on a baking sheet. Use a fork to poke holes into the sweet potatoes, set them on the baking sheet, and roast for 40 to 50 minutes, or until puffed up and soft inside when pierced with a fork.

# Day 15

Breakfast
Preparation Time: 15 Mins
Cook Time: 30 Mins
Total Time: 45 Mins
Servings: 12
Ingredients

## Chocolate Cake

- 1 3/4 cups all purpose flour, or (plain flour), (8 oz | 227 g)
- 3/4 cup unsweetened cocoa powder, (2.6 oz | 75 g) or regular Hershey's cocoa powder
- 1 1/2 teaspoon baking powder
- 1 1/2 teaspoon baking soda, (or bi-carb soda)
- 1 teaspoon salt
- 2 cups white granulated sugar, (14 oz | 410 g)
- 2 large eggs
- 1 cup milk, (250 ml)
- 1/2 cup vegetable oil, (125 ml)
- 2 teaspoons pure vanilla extract
- 1 cup boiling water (250 ml)

## Chocolate Buttercream Frosting

- 4 oz butter, (120 g | 1/2 cup)
- 2/3 cup unsweetened cocoa powder, or regular HERSHEY'S (2.4 oz | 65 g)
- 3 cups powdered sugar, (confectioners or icing sugar)
- 1/3 cup milk
- 1 teaspoon pure vanilla extract

Instructions
- Preheat oven to 350°F (180°C) standard or 320°F (160°C) fan/convection.

- Lightly grease 2x 9-inch (22cm) round cake pans with butter. Line base with parchment paper.
- Sift together flour, cocoa, baking powder, baking soda and salt into a large bowl. Whisk in sugar, then add eggs, milk, oil and vanilla. Whisk well to combine until lump free, about 30 seconds.
- Pour boiling water into batter, mixing well. Cake batter is thin in consistency.
- Pour batter into cake pans and bake for 30-35 minutes or until a wooden skewer inserted into the centre comes out clean.
- Let cool for 10 minutes, then turn out onto wire racks to cool completely before frosting.

# Lunch

## Roast Beef

Preparation Time: 15 Mins
Cook: 1 Hr
Servings: 4
Ingredients
- 1 tsp plain flour
- 1 tsp mustard powder
- 950g beef top rump joint (see tip below)
- 1 onion, cut into 8 wedges
- 500g carrots, halved lengthways

## For the Gravy

- 1 tbsp plain flour
- 250ml beef stock

Instructions
- Heat oven to 240C/220C fan/gas 9.
- Mix 1 tsp plain flour and 1 tsp mustard powder with some seasoning, then rub all over the 950g beef top rump joint.

- Put 1 onion, cut into 8 wedges, and 500g carrots, halved lengthways, into a roasting tin and sit the beef on top, then cook for 20 mins.
- Reduce oven to 190C/170C fan/gas 5 and continue to cook the beef for 30 mins if you like it rare, 40 mins for medium and 1 hr for well done.
- Remove the beef and carrots from the oven, place onto warm plates or platters and cover with foil to keep warm.
- Let the beef rest for 30 mins while you turn up the oven to cook your Yorkshire puds and finish the potatoes.
- For the gravy, put the tin with all the meat juices and onions back onto the hob.
- Stir in 1 tbsp plain flour, scraping all the stuck bits off the bottom of the tin. Cook for 30 seconds, then slowly stir in 250ml beef stock, little by little.
- Bubble to a nice gravy, season, then serve with the beef, carved into slices, carrots and all the other trimmings.

## Dinner
Preparation Time: 10 Mins
Cook: 20 Mins
Servings: 4
Ingredients
- 3 tbsp plain flour
- 4 cod loin fillets
- 2 tbsp olive oil
- 1 lemon, sliced
- ½ small bunch of thyme

Instructions
- Heat the oven to 220C/200C fan/gas 7. Tip the flour into a bowl and add some seasoning. Turn each cod fillet in the flour until evenly coated.
- Heat half the oil in a non-stick frying pan over a medium-high heat. Add the cod and fry on each side for 2 mins or until golden brown.

- Transfer the cod to a roasting tin. Arrange the lemon slices and thyme on and around the fish and drizzle with the remaining oil. Bake for 10 mins or until cooked through.

# Day 16

## Breakfast

Tomato Mozzarella Salad

Preparation time: 10 mins
Total time: 10 mins
Servings: 6
Ingredients

- 3 large tomatoes, sliced
- 8 ounces mozzarella cheese, sliced
- ¼ cup olive oil
- ¼ cup balsamic vinegar
- ¼ teaspoon salt
- ⅛ teaspoon ground black pepper
- ¼ cup minced fresh basil

Instructions

- Gather all ingredients
- Place tomato slices, alternating with mozzarella slices, on a large serving platter
- Combine oil, balsamic vinegar, salt, and pepper in a jar with a tight-fitting lid; shake well.
- Drizzle over tomatoes and mozzarella; sprinkle with basil.

## Lunch

Mexican Lasagna

Servings: 12
Ingredients

- 1 pound ground beef
- 1 medium yellow onion diced
- 2 teaspoons minced garlic 2 cloves
- 1/4 cup taco seasoning 2 packets
- 1/2 cup water
- 14.5 ounce fire roasted diced tomatoes do not drain

- 4 ounce green chiles 1 can
- 15 ounce black beans 1 can, drained and rinsed
- 18 corn tortillas
- 6 cups shredded cheese jack and cheddar
- 1 medium tomato 1-2 tomatoes diced for garnish
- 1 bunch green onions sliced for garnish
- sour cream for serving

## Instructions

- Preheat the oven to 350 degrees Fahrenheit. Spray a 9×13 casserole dish with non-stick cooking spray and set aside.
- Cook ground beef and onion in a large skillet over medium heat until the meat is browned and the onions softens.
- Add minced garlic to the skillet and saute for 1-2 minutes longer.
- Add taco seasoning and water and stir over medium heat until well combined.
- Stir the tomatoes (juices included), green chiles, and black beans into the meat mixture and heat through.
- Line the prepared baking dish with 6 corn tortillas, overlapping slightly to cover the bottom of the casserole dish.
- Spread 1/3 of the meat mixture over the tortillas. Sprinkle 2 cups of the cheese over the meat mixture.
- Continue layering corn tortillas, meat mixture, and cheese to form three layers total.
- Cover with aluminum foil and bake for 30-40 minutes until casserole is bubbly and the cheese is fully melted.
- Garnish with diced tomatoes and green onion. Let the casserole sit for 10 minutes for easy slicing and serving.
- Serve with sour cream.

# Dinner

## Potato Salad

Preparation time: 20 mins

Cook time: 20 mins
Total time: 40 mins
Ingredients
- 5 pounds Yukon Gold potatoes or Klondike Goldust potatoes
- 2 cups mayonnaise (your favorite brand)
- 1 cup refrigerated sweet pickle relish
- 2 tablespoons yellow mustard, or 1 part yellow + 1 part dijon
- 1 tablespoon apple cider vinegar
- 1 tablespoon celery seeds
- 1/2 teaspoon paprika
- 4-5 hard boiled eggs, peeled and chopped
- 3 celery stalks, diced
- 1/2 cup sweet onion, diced
- 1 tablespoon fresh chopped dill
- Salt and pepper

Instructions
- Cut the potatoes into quarters and place them in a large stockpot. Fill the pot with cold water until it is 1 inch over the top of the potatoes. Set the pot over high heat and bring to a boil. Once boiling, add 1 tablespoon salt and cook the potatoes for 13-15 minutes, until fork tender.
- Meanwhile, in a medium bowl mix the mayonnaise, sweet pickle relish including juices, mustard, apple cider vinegar, celery seeds, paprika, 1 teaspoon salt, and pepper to taste. Stir until smooth. Then chop the eggs, celery, onions, and dill.
- Once the potatoes are very tender, drain off all the water. Remove the loose peels and chop the potatoes into 1/2-inch chunks. It's okay if they are soft and crumbly. Place the potatoes in a large bowl. Gently mix in the dressing until it coats the potatoes well. Then stir in the eggs, celery, onions, and dill. Taste, then salt and pepper as needed. Garnish with fresh dill and paprika.

# Day 17

## Breakfast

BBQ Black Bean Burger

Preparation Time: 1 Hr
Cook Time: 45 Mins
Total Time: 1hr 45 Mins
Ingredients

- 1 cup cooked + cooled ?uinoa (divided // see notes for cooking instructions)
- 1 15-ounce can black beans (rinsed and dried)
- 2/3 cup raw pecans
- 1 Tbsp coconut or avocado oil (plus more for cooking burgers // or water)
- 1 heaping cup sliced and peeled sweet potato (cut into 1/4-inch rounds)
- 2 heaping cups thinly sliced cremini or button mushrooms
- 2 Tbsp coconut aminos (optional)
- 1/2 tsp sea salt (plus more to taste)
- 2 1/2 tsp chili powder
- 2 1/2 tsp cumin powder
- 3 Tbsp vegan-friendly BBQ sauce (I like Annie's organic original BBQ sauce // plus more for glazing)

For servings

- Vegan-friendly hamburger buns OR lettuce wraps (and gluten-free if needed)
- Veggies of choice (i.e. onion, cabbage, tomato, pickles)

Instructions

- If you haven't yet, cook ?uinoa and set aside to cool (see notes for instructions).
- Preheat oven to 350 degrees F (176 C) and spread rinsed, dried black beans onto a parchment-lined baking sheet.

Bake beans for 6 minutes. Then add pecans to the baking sheet and bake for 10 minutes more. The nuts should be fragrant and golden brown (be careful not to burn), and the beans should appear dry and cracked open (this way, they do not become mushy in the burger mix). Set aside to cool. Increase oven temperature to 375 degrees F (190 C).

- In the meantime, heat a medium to large cast-iron or metal skillet over medium/medium-low heat. Once hot, add oil (or water) and the sweet potato. Cover and cook for 3-4 minutes, turning heat down if the potatoes are browning too quickly. Once browned on the underside, flip and cook for 3-4 minutes more or until tender and golden brown. Remove from the pan.
- To the still-hot pan, add the sliced mushrooms and coconut aminos (optional – sub a little salt otherwise) and cook on medium/medium-high for about 4-5 minutes, stirring frequently, or until they're browned, fragrant, and cooked down to half their size. Set aside.
- To a food processor, add beans and pecans and blitz/pulse into a loose meal (some texture is good – you don't want a powder).
- Next, add cooked sweet potato, mushrooms, half the quinoa, sea salt, chili powder, cumin, and BBQ sauce and pulse a few times to combine (again, some texture is good here – you're not going for a purée).
- Transfer the mixture to a mixing bowl and stir in the rest of the quinoa. Then taste and adjust flavor as needed, adding more cumin for smokiness, chili powder for heat, BBQ sauce for sweetness / depth of flavor, or salt for saltiness.
- If the mixture appears too wet, add more quinoa. If it looks too dry, add more BBQ sauce (or a little coconut aminos) to moisten.
- Divide the mixture into four even balls and form into patties with your hands or by lining a 1/2 cup measuring cup with plastic wrap, packing the mixture inside, then lifting the plastic wrap out – mash slightly into more of a disc. Refrigerate burgers for 30 minutes.

- Once chilled, heat the cast-iron or metal pan from earlier over medium heat. Once hot, add a bit more oil (or water) and the burgers. Cook for 4-5 minutes. Then carefully flip and cook for 4-5 minutes on the other side. Then turn off heat, glaze/brush with a bit more BBQ sauce, and transfer the pan to the oven. Bake at 375 F (190C) for 10-15 minutes more. The burgers should appear browned.
- Serve as is or with toppings. We enjoyed ours on buns with butter lettuce, shredded red pepper, shredded cabbage, pickles, radish, and more BBQ sauce. Store leftovers in the refrigerator for 3-4 days or in the freezer up to 1 month

# Lunch

## Chicken Paprikash

Preparation Time: 10 Mins
Cook Time: 40 Mins
Total Time: 50 Mins
Servings: 4-6
Ingredients
- 2 to 2 1/2 pounds chicken pieces, preferably thighs and drumsticks
- Kosher salt
- 2 to 3 tablespoons unsalted butter
- 2 pounds yellow onions (about 2 to 3 large onions)
- Freshly ground black pepper to taste
- 2 tablespoons sweet paprika, preferably Hungarian
- 1 teaspoon hot paprika or cayenne, or to taste
- 1 cup chicken broth
- 1/2 cup sour cream

Instructions
- Sprinkle the chicken well with salt and set aside at room temperature.
- Slice the onions lengthwise (top to root).
- Heat a large sauté pan over medium-high heat and melt the butter. When the butter is hot, pat the chicken pieces dry

with paper towels and place them skin-side down in the pan. Let the chicken pieces cook 4 to 5 minutes on one side, until well browned, then turn them over and let them cook 2 to 3 minutes on the other side. (Take care when turning so as not to tear the skin if any is sticking to the pan.)

- Remove the chicken from the pan to a bowl, set aside.
- Add the sliced onions to the sauté pan and cook them, stirring occasionally, scraping up the browned bits from the chicken, until lightly browned, about 7 minutes.
- Add the paprika and black pepper to the onions and stir to combine. Let cook for a minute.
- Add the chicken broth, again scraping up the browned bits from the bottom of the pan, and then nestle the chicken pieces into the pan, on top of the onions. Cover and cook on a low simmer for 20 to 25 minutes (depending on the size of your chicken pieces).
- When the chicken is cooked through to 165°F, (use a digital thermometer) remove the pan from the heat.
- When the chicken is done to your taste, remove the chicken from the pan. Allow the pan to cool for a minute and then slowly stir in the sour cream and add salt to taste.
- If the sour cream cools the sauce too much, turn the heat back on just enough to warm it through. Add the chicken back to the pan and coat with the sauce.
- Serve with dumplings, rice, egg noodles or potatoes. (If cooking gluten-free, serve with rice, potatoes or gluten-free noodles or dumplings.)

## Dinner

## Fried Apple

Preparation Time: 10 Mins
Cook Time: 20 Mins
Servings: 6
Ingredients
- ½ cup butter

- 6 apples (Granny Smith)
- ½ cup granulated white sugar (granulated, white)
- ¼ cup brown sugar (packed)
- 1 teaspoon cinnamon
- 1 pinch nutmeg
- 1 pinch salt

## Instructions

### Get prepped

- Peel, core and slice the apples into even pieces.

### Cook the Apples

- Melt the butter in a large skillet over medium heat.
- Add the apples, cover, and cook over low heat for 15-20 minutes, until the apples are soft. Stir often so they don't burn.

### Add remaining ingredients

- Mix the white sugar, brown sugar, cinnamon, nutmeg and salt together in a bowl.
- Add to the apples and stir. Cook for another 5-10 minutes until the sugar is dissolved and are syrupy.
- Serve over ice-cream, or as a side.

# Day 18

## Breakfast

### Chinese Spareribs

Preparation Time: 5 Mins
Cook Time: 40 Mins
Additional Time: 2 Hrs
Total Time: 2hrs 45 Mins
Servings: 2
Ingredients
- 3 tablespoons hoisin sauce
- 1 tablespoon ketchup
- 1 tablespoon honey
- 1 tablespoon soy sauce
- 1 tablespoon sake
- 1 teaspoon rice vinegar
- 1 teaspoon lemon juice
- 1 teaspoon grated fresh ginger
- ½ teaspoon grated fresh garlic
- ¼ teaspoon Chinese five-spice powder
- 1 pound pork spareribs

Instructions
- Mix together hoisin sauce, ketchup, honey, soy sauce, sake, rice vinegar, lemon juice, ginger, garlic, and five-spice powder in a shallow glass dish. Place ribs in the dish and turn to coat. Cover and marinate in the refrigerator for 2 hours or up to overnight.
- Preheat the oven to 325 degrees F (165 degrees C). Fill a broiler tray with enough water to cover the bottom. Place the grate or a rack over the tray; arrange ribs on the grate.
- Cook in the preheated oven on the center rack for 40 minutes, turning and brushing with marinade every 10 minutes. Let marinade cook on for final 10 minutes to

make a glaze. Finish under the broiler if desired. Discard any remaining marinade.

# Lunch

## Chicken Salad

Preparation Time: 10 Mins
Poaching Chicken: 20 Mins
Total Time: 30 Mins
Servings: 4
Ingredients

For the Salad:

- 1 pound raw boneless, skinless chicken breasts, cut into 2 1/2-inch chunks (or 2 to 3 cups cooked chicken meat)
- 2 ribs celery, chopped
- 1/2 red bell pepper, seeded and chopped
- 4 to 6 green olives, pitted and minced
- 1/4 cup chopped red onion
- 1/2 to 1 apple, cored and chopped
- 1/3 head iceberg lettuce, sliced and chopped

For the dressing:

- 5 tablespoons mayonnaise
- 1 tablespoon plum preserves, or any sweet berry preserve (or a lesser amount of honey)
- 2 teaspoons freshly squeezed lemon juice
- Salt and pepper to taste

Instructions
- Bring a pot with 2 quarts of well salted water (1 tablespoon salt) to a boil. Add the chicken breast (cut into large chunks) and return the water to a simmer. Then turn off the heat, and cover the pot. Let the chicken sit for 15

minutes (time it) or more while you prepare everything else.
- Prepare the chicken salad dressing in a large bowl. Mix together the mayonnaise, preserves, and lemon juice. Taste for the proper balance of sweetness and acidity. The salad dressing should not be too sweet, nor too sour.
- Add more preserves or lemon juice until you have reached the balance you want. Add salt and pepper to taste.
- Mix in the chopped celery, bell pepper, olives, red onion, and apple
- Remove the chicken from the poaching water and dice it. (Or dice already cooked chicken if that is what you are using for this salad.) Mix it in with the dressing and vegetables.
- At this point you can make ahead. When ready to serve, fold in the sliced and chopped iceberg lettuce.

## Dinner

Farro Bowl

Preparation Time: 15 Mins
Cook Time: 25 Mins
Total Time: 40 Mins
Servings: 4
Ingredients
- 1cup (200 g) uncooked farro
- 4-5 cups (200g) finely chopped kale
- 1 cup(150g) diced red onion
- 2 red bell peppers
- 1 cup(240g) drained and rinsed chickpeas, or more if desired
- 32 kalamata olives, or more if desired
- 1 cup (50g) lightly packed, finely chopped parsley
- For the lemon tahini sauce
- 6 tbsp (90 g) tahini
- ¼ cup(60ml) water

- 3 cloves garlic, grated
- 2 tsp(10ml) maple syrup
- 1 tsp salt

Instructions
- Cook the farro according to package instructions.
- While the farro is cooking, make the roasted red peppers. Find complete instructions for roasted red peppers here (no other ingredients required).
- Prepare the dressing by blending all of the ingredients together until smooth, start with 1/4 cup of water and add a splash more at a time if needed to adjust the consistency. It should be thick and creamy but easy to drizzle.
- To prepare the kale, give it a good wash then tear the leaves away from the stems. Finely chop the leaves and either add 1/4 tsp olive or or a squeeze of lemon and massage and squeeze the kale for 1-2 minutes until softened.
- To assemble the bowls, divide the kale between 4 servings then top each with equal amounts of the other ingredients. Drizzle with tahini dressing.

# Day 19

## Breakfast

Grilled Vegetable

Preparation Time: 9 Mins
Cook Time: 16 Mins
Total Time: 25 Mins
Serving: 4
Ingredients
- 1 yellow squash
- 1 zucchini
- 8 ounces cremini mushrooms, stemmed
- 1 small red onion
- 1 red bell pepper
- 1 green bell pepper
- 1 ear fresh corn, cut into 1-inch rounds
- Extra virgin olive oil, for drizzling
- Sea salt and freshly ground black pepper
- tzatziki, pesto, or Greek dressing for drizzling/serving

Instructions
- Heat a grill to medium-high and spray with nonstick cooking spray. Cut the vegetables into similar sized chunks and thread onto 4 metal skewers. Drizzle with olive oil and season with salt and pepper. Grill the skewers for 8 minutes per side or until the vegetables are tender and lightly charred. Remove from the grill, season to taste, and serve with desired sauce or dressing.

## Lunch

Creamy Hot Cheese Dip

Total Time: 30minutes
Servings: 4-6
Ingredients

- 8 oz 225gr American cheese slices
- 4 oz 115gr Cheddar & Monterey Jack cheese (or just cheddar cheese), cubed or grated
- 2/3 cup 160ml milk (I used whole milk, but any will work)
- 1/3 cup 80ml heavy whipping cream
- 3 tablespoons chopped canned jalapenos
- 2-3 tablespoons canned jalapeno juice
- ¼ teaspoon ground cumin
- ¼ teaspoon cayenne pepper
- ¼ teaspoon chili pepper

Instructions
- In a medium saucepan, place the cheese and melt on low heat.
- Stir in milk and heavy cream, whisking continuously until smooth.
- Add chopped jalapenos, jalapeno juice, and seasonings.
- Serve hot with some good tortilla chips.

# Dinner

## Corn on the Cob

Preparation Time: 5 Mins
Cook Time: 8 Mins
Total: 13 Minutes
Servings: 6-8
Ingredients
- 6-8 ears of corn, husks and silks removed and cut in half (if desired)
- 1 cup milk
- 1 stick Challenge butter

Instructions
- Fill a large pot about halfway with water.
- Bring water to a boil.
- Add milk and butter. Add corn and reduce heat.
- Simmer corn for 6 to 8 minutes.

- Remove corn from cooking liquid and its ready to serve.

# Day 20

## Breakfast

### Kidney Bean Salad

Preparation time: 10 minutes
Cook time: 0 minute
Total time: 10 minutes
Servings: 6
Ingredients

#### For the Salad

- 1½ cups (1 x 15oz can) kidney beans , drained and rinsed, (a 398 ml can in Canada)
- 1½ cups (1 x 15oz can) chickpeas , drained and rinsed, (a 398 ml can in Canada)
- 1 medium cucumber , diced
- ½ medium sweet white or red onion , finely chopped
- 1 cup (or 1 to 2 big handfuls) flat leaf parsley , chopped or torn

#### For the Dressing

- 5 tablespoons fresh lemon juice , usually around 1 large juicy lemon or 1½ medium ones
- 3 tablespoons extra virgin olive oil , (omit to make oil-free)
- 2 small cloves garlic , minced very finely or grated
- 1 - 2 teaspoons sugar , or a little drop of maple syrup or agave
- ½ teaspoon salt , or to taste
- ½ teaspoon freshly cracked black pepper , or to taste

### Instructions
- Drain and rinse the beans then add to a large salad bowl.
- Add the chopped cucumber, onion and parsley.

- Whisk all of the dressing ingredients together, or put them in a jar and give them a good shake. I recommend adding the sugar to taste so you get the perfect balance of tangy and sweet for you.
- Pour the dressing over the salad and toss together well.

# Lunch

## Oatmeal Cookies

Preparation Time: 15 Minutes
Cook Time: 10 Minutes
Additional Time: 1hr 15 Mins
Total Time: 1hr 30 Mins
Servings: 24
Ingredients
- 2 cups all-purpose flour
- 1 ½ teaspoons ground cinnamon
- 1 teaspoon baking soda
- 1 teaspoon salt
- 1 cup unsalted butter, softened
- 1 cup white sugar
- 1 cup packed brown sugar
- 2 large eggs
- 1 teaspoon vanilla extract
- 3 cups quick cooking oats
- nonstick cooking spray with flour
- 2 tablespoons water
- 2 tablespoons white sugar, or as needed

Instructions
- Whisk flour, cinnamon, baking soda, and salt together in a medium bowl until well combined.
- Beat butter, 1 cup white sugar, and brown sugar in a large bowl with an electric mixer until creamy, at least 2 to 3 minutes. Beat in eggs, one at a time, then mix in vanilla. Gradually mix in dry ingredients until well combined. Add

oats and mix until thoroughly incorporated. Cover the bowl and chill dough in the refrigerator for at least 1 hour.

- When ready to bake, preheat the oven to 375 degrees F (190 degrees C). Spray two cookie sheets with floured cooking spray. Place water in a small bowl and 2 tablespoons sugar in another small bowl.
- Roll chilled dough into walnut-sized balls, and place 2 inches apart on the prepared cookie sheets. Dip a large fork in water, then in sugar, and use to flatten each cookie, rewetting and resugaring as necessary.
- Bake in the preheated oven until light golden brown around the edges and centers are nearly set, 8 to 10 minutes, switching racks halfway through. Allow cookies to cool on baking sheet for 5 minutes before transferring to a wire rack to cool completely.

# Dinner

## Zucchini Boats

Preparation time: 10 mins
Cook time: 40 mins
Total time: 50 mins
Ingredients
- 4 medium zucchini
- 1/2 teaspoon dried Italian seasoning
- salt and pepper to taste
- 2 teaspoons olive oil
- 1 pound mild Italian sausage casings removed
- 1/2 cup onion finely diced
- 1 teaspoon minced garlic
- 2 cups marinara sauce
- 3/4 cup shredded mozzarella cheese
- 1 tablespoon chopped parsley
- cooking spray

## Instructions

- Preheat the oven to 400 degrees F. Coat a large rectangular baking with with cooking spray.
- Cut the zucchini in half lengthwise, then trim off the stem ends. Use a spoon to carefully scoop the flesh out of the zucchinis.
- Sprinkle the Italian seasoning, salt and pepper over the zucchini shells. Arrange the zucchini in the baking dish.
- Heat the olive oil in a large pan over medium high heat. Add the sausage and cook for 4-5 minutes, breaking up the meat with a spatula.
- Add the onion and cook for an additional 4 minutes or until onion is softened. Add the garlic and cook for 30 seconds.
- Season the sausage and vegetable mixture with salt and pepper.
- Pour the marinara sauce into the pan and bring to a simmer; cook for 5 minutes.
- Spoon the meat mixture evenly into the zucchini shells, then top with the shredded cheese.
- Bake for 25 minutes, or until zucchini is tender and cheese is melted and golden brown.
- Sprinkle with parsley, then serve.

# Day 21

## Breakfast

## Palak Tofu

Preparation Time: 15 Mins
Cook Time: 20 Mins
Total Time: 35 Mins
Servings: 4
Ingredients
- 6 oz extra-firm tofu cut into cubes
- 2 teaspoons oil
- 1/8 teaspoon ground pepper
- 1/8 teaspoon smoked paprika
- 1/8 teaspoon red chili flakes
- salt to taste
- spinach curry
- 1 lb baby spinach
- 2 tomatoes roughly chopped
- 3-4 garlic cloves roughly chopped
- 1 inch ginger roughly chopped
- 1/2 teaspoon garam masala to sprinkle
- 1/8 teaspoon red chili powder or to taste
- 3/4 teaspoon cumin powder
- 1/2 cup coconut milk or substitute with milk or heavy cream
- 2.5 teaspoons oil
- salt to taste
- 1-2 teaspoon sugar or honey optional
- 1 teaspoon fresh lemon juice optional

Instructions
- In a pan heat 2 teaspoons of oil. Once the oil is hot, add cubed tofu and sprinkle paprika, salt, pepper and red chilli flakes.

- Saute for 5-6 minutes till tofu is light golden brown in color. Set aside.
- Spinach Curry
- Heat 1 teaspoon of oil and cook the baby spinach till it's completely wilted. Set aside.
- In another pan, heat 1.5 teaspoon of oil on medium heat. Once hot, add roughly chopped ginger & garlic to it and saute till raw smell goes away.
- Add cubed tomatoes next and cook till tomatoes are soft and mushy, around 3-4 minutes.
- Add the wilted spinach leaves and also add cumin powder, red chilli powder, salt and garam masala.
- Cook the spinach and tomato with the spices for 2 minutes.
- Remove from heat, let it cool down a bit and then transfer mixture to a blender.
- Add 1/4 cup of milk/coconut milk and grind to a smooth paste. Set aside.
- Take the same pan in which you had cooked the tomato and spinach and add the spinach puree to it on medium heat. Add additional 1/4 cup milk/coconut milk and mix.
- Add the sauteed tofu to the spinach curry.
- Mix well and also add water at this step [if re?uired] to adjust the consistency of curry to preference.
- Add sugar/honey [if using] and mix.
- Cover and let the curry simmer for 10 minutes on medium-low heat.
- Squeeze in some fresh lemon juice (optional) and serve hot with Indian bread or rice!.

# Lunch

## Asian Asparagus

Preparation Time: 15 Minutes
Servings: 6
Ingredients

- 1 ½lbs fresh asparagus, washed,hard stems snapped off,if necessary peel the bottom part of the stem
- 2teaspoons vegetable oil
- ¼cup water
- 1pinch sugar
- 2cloves garlic, minced
- 1teaspoon sesame seed oil
- 1tablespoon reduced sodium soy sauce
- 1tablespoon oyster sauce
- 1tablespoon dry sherry
- 2teaspoons rice wine vinegar
- ¼teaspoon crushed red pepper flakes
- 2tablespoons green onions, chopped (white & green part)

Instructions
- Cut asparagus into 2" pieces.
- Heat oil in wok or large skillet (high heat).
- Add asparagus, stir fry for 1 minute.
- Add water& sugar to the asparagus, cover and steam for 2 minutes, shake the pan a few times Combine the remaining ingredients.
- Uncover wok and add remaining ingredients and cook for 1 minute, stirring to coat the asparagus with the spice mixture.
- Serve immediately.

# Dinner

## Couscous Salad

Preparation Time: 25 Minutes
Cook Time: 5 Minutes
Ingredients
- 1 cup dry Moroccan couscous*
- 1 cup warm water**
- Salt and freshly ground black pepper
- 1/4 cup + 1 tsp olive oil, divided (regular or extra virgin)

- 2 Tbsp fresh lemon juice
- 1 tsp minced garlic (1 clove)
- 1 1/2 cups grape tomatoes, halved
- 1 1/2 cups diced English cucumber
- 1/3 cup diced red onion
- 1/3 cup finely crumbled feta cheese
- 1/3 cup toasted slivered almonds (optional but highly recommended)
- 1/3 cup finely chopped fresh parsley
- 2 Tbsp finely chopped fresh mint

Instructions
- Bring water to a boil in a medium saucepan.
- Right when it reaches a boil remove from heat and right away stir in couscous and salt and cover. Let rest 5 minutes.
- Drizzle in 1 tsp olive oil, fluff with a fork and let cool about 10 minutes in a salad bowl (toss occasionally if possible to reduce sticking). Meanwhile prepare remaining salad ingredients.
- In a small mixing bowl whisk together remaining 1/4 cup olive oil, lemon juice and garlic.
- To bowl with couscous add tomatoes, cucumber, red onion, feta, almonds if using, parsley, and mint. Pour dressing over everything and toss to evenly coat.
- Season with salt and pepper to taste. Salad is best the day prepared but will keep in the fridge for 1 day.

# Day 22

## Breakfast

Creamy Turkey Casserole

Preparation Time: 20 Mins
Cook Time: 50 Mins
Total Time: 1hrs 10 Mins
Servings: 6
Ingredients
- 3 cups uncooked penne or medium pasta
- 3 tablespoons butter
- 1 onion finely diced
- 8 ounces mushrooms sliced
- 2 cloves garlic minced
- 10 ¾ ounces condensed cream of chicken soup
- 1 ⅓ cups milk
- ½ teaspoon seasoned salt
- ½ teaspoon dried basil
- 1 cup havarti cheese or swiss cheese, shredded
- 3 cups cooked turkey

## Topping

- ¼ cup seasoned bread crumbs
- 2 tablespoons butter melted
- Instructions
- Heat oven to 375°F. Combine topping ingredients and set aside.
- Cook pasta al dente according to package directions.
- Cook onion, mushrooms, and garlic in butter until tender, about 5 minutes.
- In a large bowl combine soup, mushroom mixture, milk, seasonings, and ½ of the cheese. Fold in turkey and pasta.
- Spread into a 9x13 casserole dish, top with remaining cheese, and sprinkle with topping.

- Bake 30-35 minutes or until hot and bubbly.

# Lunch

## Vegetarian Chili

Preparation Time: 10 Mins
Total Time: 1hr
Servings: 6-8 Servings
Ingredients
- 1 tbsp. extra-virgin olive oil
- 1 medium yellow onion, chopped
- 1 red bell pepper, chopped
- 2 carrots, peeled and finely chopped
- 3 cloves garlic, minced
- 1 jalapeño, finely chopped
- 1 tbsp. tomato paste
- 1 (15.5-oz.) can pinto beans, drained and rinsed
- 1 (15.5-oz.) can black beans, drained and rinsed
- 1 (15.5-oz.) can kidney beans, drained and rinsed
- 1 (28-oz.) can fire roasted tomatoes
- 3 c. low-sodium vegetable broth
- 2 tbsp. chili powder
- 1 tbsp. ground cumin
- 2 tsp. dried oregano
- Kosher salt
- Freshly ground black pepper
- Shredded cheddar, for serving
- Sour cream, for serving
- Cilantro, for serving

Instructions
- In a large pot over medium heat, heat olive oil. Add onion, bell pepper, and carrots. Sauté until soft, about 5 minutes. Add garlic and jalapeño and cook until fragrant, 1 minute.

- Add tomato paste and stir to coat vegetables. Add tomatoes, beans, broth, and seasonings. Season with salt and pepper to taste.
- Bring to a boil then reduce heat and let simmer, 30 minutes.
- Serve with cheese, sour cream, and cilantro.

## Dinner

### Pecan And Parmesan Crusted Tilapia

Preparation Time: 15 Mins
Total 30 Mins
Servings: 4
Servings: 4
Ingredients
- 1 lbs. asparagus, trimmed
- 1 tbsp. Gustare Vita olive oil
- 1 tsp. lemon zest
- ½ tsp. kosher salt, divided
- ½ tsp. coarse-ground black pepper
- 1 lemon, sliced
- 4 (4-to 6-oz.) fresh Rainforest tilapia fillets
- ½ c. Hy-Vee mayonnaise
- 2 tbsp. Weber honey-garlic rub, divided
- ⅔ c. Hy-Vee chopped pecans
- ¼ c. Soirée grated Parmesan cheese
- 2 tbsp. Hy-Vee plain panko bread crumbs
- Fresh thyme, for garnish

Instructions
- Preheat oven to 425 degrees. Line 2 baking sheets with foil and spray with nonstick spray; set aside.
- Place asparagus on one prepared sheet. Drizzle with olive oil; toss to coat. Sprinkle with lemon zest, 1/4 teaspoon salt, and pepper. Add lemon slices.

- pat tilapia dry with paper towels. Stir together mayonnaise and 1 tablespoon honey-garlic rub in a small bowl; set aside. Combine chopped pecans, Parmesan cheese, bread crumbs, and remaining 1 tablespoon honey garlic rub in another small bowl.
- Spread mayonnaise mixture on top of fish fillets. Generously sprinkle with pecan mixture; press to adhere. Place fish on remaining prepared baking sheet; lightly spray with nonstick spray.
- Bake fish and asparagus with lemons 16 to 18 minutes or until coating is golden brown and fish reaches 145 degrees, and asparagus is fork-tender. Garnish with fresh thyme, if desired.

# Day 23

## Breakfast

### Cucumber Sandwich

Active Time: 10 Mins
Total Time: 10 Mins
Servings: 1
Ingredients
- 2 ounces cream cheese, at room temperature
- 1 tablespoon low-fat plain Greek yogurt
- 1 tablespoon sliced fresh chives
- 1 tablespoon chopped fresh dill
- ¼ teaspoon ground pepper
- 2 slices whole-wheat sandwich bread
- ⅓ cup thinly sliced English cucumber

Instructions
- Stir cream cheese, yogurt, chives, dill and pepper together in a small bowl until well blended. Spread the mixture evenly on one side of each bread slice. Top 1 slice with cucumber slices, then top with the other bread slice, cream cheese-side down. Cut the crusts from the sandwich and cut it in half diagonally.

## Lunch

### Spanish Bean Soup

Preparation Time: 40 Mins
Cook Time: 1hr 30 Mins
Total Time: 2hr 10 Mins
Ingredients
- 1 pound dried Garbanzo (chickpea) beans
- 1 spoon of olive oil
- 1 tablespoon salt
- 2 potatoes

- 1 large onion (or 2 small)
- 6 cups of water
- ½ teaspoon ground black pepper
- 2 Chorizos (Spanish sausage)
- 3 ounces chicken stock
- 2 cloves Garlic (minced)
- ½ pound smoked ham
- 2 teaspoons saffron yellow (optional)
- 1 teaspoon paprika (optional)
- 1 ham bone (optional)
- Spices: fresh chopped thyme, rosemary, oregano, and ground cumin

Instructions
- Wash and rinse the Garbanzo beans in a large bowl, cover them with water and a tablespoon of salt, then let it soak overnight. Or you can boil them on medium heat for 30 minutes to one hour.
- Meanwhile cut the Chorizo, garlic, onions, and ham into cubes or any shape of your choice. Place them on a large pot with enough chicken stock to cover them (about two inches). Cook for 30 minutes.
- Cut the potatoes in quarters.
- After that pour the beans (strained), spices, and the remaining stock. Cook for 30 more minutes removing any foam.
- Add the potatoes and cook for 30 more minutes. Taste a little bit to see if it needs more salt.
- Serve warm and enjoy!

# Dinner

## Carrot Soup

Active Time: 40 Mins
Additional Time: 10 Mins
Total Time: 50 Mins

Servings: 8
Ingredients
- 1 tablespoon butter
- 1 tablespoon extra-virgin olive oil
- 1 medium onion, chopped
- 1 stalk celery, chopped
- 2 cloves garlic, chopped
- 1 teaspoon chopped fresh thyme or parsley
- 5 cups chopped carrots
- 2 cups water
- 4 cups reduced-sodium chicken broth, "no-chicken" broth (see Note) or vegetable broth
- ½ cup half-and-half (optional)
- ½ teaspoon salt
- Freshly ground pepper to taste

Instructions
- Heat butter and oil in a Dutch oven over medium heat until the butter melts. Add onion and celery; cook, stirring occasionally, until softened, 4 to 6 minutes. Add garlic and thyme (or parsley); cook, stirring, until fragrant, about 10 seconds. Stir in carrots. Add water and broth; bring to a lively simmer over high heat. Reduce heat to maintain a lively simmer and cook until very tender, about 25 minutes.
- Puree the soup in batches in a blender until smooth. (Use caution when pureeing hot li uids.) Stir in half-and-half (if using), salt and pepper.

# Day 24

## Breakfast

Avocado Lime Slaw

Preparation time: 10 mins
Total time: 10 mins
Servings: 6
Ingredients
- ½ cup mayonnaise
- 1 avocado pit and skin removed, sliced in half
- ½ cup cilantro roughly chopped
- 2 cloves garlic minced
- 3 tbsp lime juice fresh
- 1 jalapeno seeded and finely chopped
- ½ tsp Kosher salt
- ¼ tsp black pepper freshly ground
- 12 oz slaw mix

Instructions
- In a food processor, add mayonnaise, avocado, cilantro, garlic, lime juice, jalapeno, salt, and pepper. Pulse until completely blended and smooth.
- Place the slaw mix in a large bowl and spoon the dressing over the top. Use two large spoons to toss the slaw until fully mixed.
- Serve at once, or cover and place in the fridge for up to 24 hours.

## Lunch

Basic Pie Dough

Preparation Time: 10 Mins
Total Time: 2 Hrs 10 Mins
Ingredients
- 2 1/2 c. all-purpose flour, spooned and leveled

- 1 tsp. Kosher salt
- 1 tsp. sugar
- 1 c. cold unsalted butter, cut up
- 1/4 c. ice water

## Instructions

- Whisk together flour, salt, and sugar. Cut in butter until it resembles coarse meal with several pea-size pieces remaining. Add water, 1 tablespoon at a time, using a fork to pull dough together into a crumbly pile (add up to an additional 2 tablespoons of water if needed).
- Divided dough into two piles; wrap each in plastic wrap. Use the plastic to flatten and press dough into disks. Refrigerate until firm, 2 hours.
- Bring dough to room temperature and roll out on a counter or cutting board lightly dusted with flour until 1/8 inch thick. Then press into pan and par-bake or fill as pie recipe instructs.

## Dinner

## Chicken in Wine

Preparation Time: 15 Mins
Cook Time: 25 Mins
Servings: 4
Ingredients

- 2 (12 oz) boneless skinless chicken breasts
- Salt and freshly ground black pepper
- 1/3 cup all-purpose flour
- 1 Tbsp olive oil
- 4 Tbsp Danish Creamery European Style Unsalted Butter, cut into 1 Tbsp pieces, divided
- 1 cup finely chopped yellow onion (1 small)
- 2 tsp minced garlic (2 cloves)
- 1 1/2 cups + 1 Tbsp low-sodium chicken broth, divided
- 1 cup dry white wine, recommend Sauvigon Blanc
- 2 tsp thyme leaves

- 1.5 tsp cornstarch
- 1 Tbsp minced fresh parsley

Instructions
- Slice chicken breasts in half through the thickness to create 4 portions total. Cover with plastic wrap and pound with a meat mallet to even out their thickness.
- Heat oil in a 12-inch skillet over medium-high heat.
- Place flour in a shallow dish. Season both sides of chicken breast portions with salt and pepper then dredge each side in flour, gently shake off excess flour.
- Place chicken in skillet (spacing evenly apart) and cook until browned and cooked through, about 4 to 5 minutes per side (chicken should register 165 degrees in center of thickest portion). Note that if skillet seems dry when you turn chicken to second side then drizzle in an additional 1/2 Tbsp olive oil.
- Transfer chicken to a plate and cover with aluminum foil to keep warm.
- Return skillet to medium heat. Add 2 Tbsp butter and stir to melt.
- Add onions and saute until tender and golden brown, about 5 minutes. Add garlic and saute 30 seconds longer.
- Slowly pour in 1 1/2 cups chicken broth and the white wine while scraping up browned bits from the bottom of the pan. Stir in thyme leaves.
- Bring to a simmer, then reduce heat to medium-low and let simmer until alcohol flavor has cooked off and sauce has reduced to about 1/3 it's original volume, about 12 - 15 minutes.
- In a small bowl whisk together remaining 1 Tbsp chicken broth with cornstarch until smooth. Once sauce in skillet has reduced stir in the cornstarch mixture and cook until thickened, while whisking, about 1 minute longer.
- Melt remaining 2 Tbsp butter in sauce. Season sauce with salt if needed and pepper to taste.

- Return chicken to sauce in skillet, spoon sauce over and sprinkle with parsley and serve.

# Day 25

Breakfast

Baked Scallops

Preparation Time: 5 Mins
Cook Time: 10 Mins
Total Time: 15 Mins
Ingredients
- 1 lb sea scallops side muscle removed
- 2 tablespoons unsalted butter melted and slightly cooled
- old bay seasoning to taste
- 1 lemon

Instructions
- Preheat your oven to 400 degrees F. and line a baking sheet with parchment paper.
- Discard the small side muscle from each scallop and pat dry the scallops on both sides with a paper towel.
- Brush each scallop with melted butter and squeeze a little bit of lemon juice over each scallop. Do this on both sides.
- Season the scallops lightly on both sides with old bay seasoning.
- Bake for 10-12 minutes or until the scallops reach an internal temperature of 125-130 degrees.
- Serve with lemon wedges and garnish with fresh parsley if desired.

Lunch

Blackened Salmon

Preparation Time: 10 Mins
Cook Time: 10 Mins
Total Time: 20 Mins
Servings: 4
Ingredients

- 4 6-ounce salmon fillet portions skin-on
- 1 tablespoon paprika
- 1 teaspoon light or dark brown sugar
- 1 teaspoon kosher salt
- 3/4 teaspoon onion powder
- 3/4 teaspoon garlic powder
- ½ teaspoon cayenne pepper
- 1/2 teaspoon dried oregano
- ½ teaspoon dried thyme
- 2 tablespoons unsalted butter
- 1 lemon cut into wedges
- Chopped fresh parsley or thyme for serving

Instructions
- Place the salmon on a large plate, flesh-side up, and pat dry.
- In a small bowl, stir together the paprika, brown sugar, salt, onion powder, garlic powder, cayenne, thyme and oregano.
- In a separate small bowl, melt the butter. Brush the butter over the flesh-side of the salmon fillets, then sprinkle the flesh sides evenly with the spice mixture. Lightly pat the spices to adhere as needed.
- Heat a large cast iron skillet or similar heavy-bottomed pan over medium heat (no need to add oil). Turn on the exhaust fan and open a window if things start to get smoky. Once the pan is completely hot (a droplet of water should dance on its surface), working quickly but gently, add the salmon fillets, one at a time, flesh-side down. Cook for 2 to 3 minutes without disturbing the fillets, until the surface is blackened (peek as little as possible so that the salmon gets a nice dark color), then carefully turn each piece of salmon over.
- Continue cooking over medium heat, until the skin becomes crispy, and the fish is fully cooked through, about 5 to 6 additional minutes depending upon the thickness of your fillets. The fish should reach 145 degrees F on an

instant read thermometer and flake easily with a fork at its thickest part.

- Squeeze lemon over the salmon, then transfer the fillets to serving plates. Serve immediately with a sprinkle of fresh thyme and additional lemon wedges.

# Dinner

## Cajun Salmon

Cook Time: 10 Mins
Preparation Time: 5 Minutes
Total Time: 15 Mins
Servings: 4
Ingredients
- 500 g (1lb) salmon fillets
- 1 tbsp olive oil
- 2 tbsp Cajun seasoning

## For the Sauce

- 1 tbsp butter
- 4 garlic cloves crushed
- ½ tsp chilli flakes
- 2 tbsp parsley finely chopped
- 1 tsp dill finely chopped
- 1 tsp thyme
- 1 cup cream
- 1 tsp lemon juice
- salt and pepper to taste

Instructions
- Pat the salmon fillets dry with paper towel. Drizzle over the olive oil then season generously with Cajun seasoning, salt and pepper.
- Heat a large frying pan over medium high heat.
- Add the salmon, skin-side down, and cook for 2-3 minutes until the skin is crisp.

- Flip over and cook for another 2-3 minutes on the other side. Remove from the pan and set aside while you make the sauce.
- In the same pan you cooked the salmon, melt the butter then add the garlic and herbs.
- Sauté for a few minutes until fragrant then pour in the cream and lemon juice.
- Allow to simmer for a few minutes then season with salt and pepper.
- Add the salmon back to the sauce and allow to simmer for another 2 minutes. Serve immediately.

# Day 26

## Breakfast

### Chicken Nuggets

Preparation Time: 20 Mins
Cook Time: 10 – 15 Minutes
Servings: 4
Ingredients
- 400g chicken breast fillets
- 4 tablespoon plain flour
- 1 egg, lightly beaten
- 115g panko breadcrumbs or other dried breadcrumbs
- 2 tablespoon vegetable or sunflower oil.

Instructions
- Cut the chicken into bite-sized pieces. Put the pieces on a layer of cling film, cover with another layer of cling film, then use a rolling pin to bash the pieces until around 2-3mm thick and uniform.
- You can either cook the chicken nuggets in a frying pan or in the oven. If you're not pan-frying, heat the oven to 220C/200C fan/gas 7 and lightly oil two baking trays.
- Tip the flour onto a plate and mix with a pinch of salt. Put the beaten egg in a bowl, and tip the breadcrumbs into another bowl.
- Dip each chicken piece in the flour, then into the egg (shaking off the excess), and finally toss in the breadcrumbs and transfer to the lightly oiled baking tray. We find that breadcrumbing using one hand is less messy.
- If cooking the nuggets in the oven, bake for 10-15 mins, turning halfway through. If pan-frying, heat the oil in a large frying pan over a high heat and cook the nuggets in two or three batches for 3-4 mins on each side until golden. carefully remove with a slotted spoon. Serve with tomato sauce, if you like.

# Lunch

## Candied Peanuts

Preparation Time: 15 Minutes
Cook Time: 20 Minutes
Total Time: 35 Minutes
Servings: 4
Ingredients
- 1 cup sugar
- 1/2 cup water
- 2 cups peanuts raw, skin on

Instructions
- Preheat oven to 300. In a medium saucepan, combine sugar and water. Place over medium heat and stir until sugar dissolves.
- 1 cup sugar,1/2 cup water
- Add peanuts to sugar water. Continue to cook over medium heat, stirring constantly, until the peanuts are completely sugar-coated and no sugar syrup remains. This will take about 30 minutes.2 cups peanuts
- Pour the boiled peanuts out onto an ungreased cookie sheet and spread them out a bit. Bake for 30 minutes, stirring every 10 minutes. Allow the roasted peanuts to cool on the cookie sheet and then store in a sealed container.

# Dinner

## Baked Scallops

Preparation time: 10 mins
Total time: 10 mins
Servings: 4
Ingredients
- 1 lb. scallops
- Kosher salt
- Freshly ground black pepper

- 4 tbsp. butter, melted
- 3 cloves garlic, minced
- Juice of 1/2 a lemon
- 1/4 c. panko bread crumbs
- 1/4 c. freshly grated Parmesan
- 4 tsp. extra-virgin olive oil
- Pinch red pepper flakes
- Lemon wedges, for serving

Instructions
- Preheat oven to 425°. Pat scallops dry with paper towels and place in a small baking dish. Season with salt and pepper.
- In a small bowl, combine melted butter, garlic, and lemon juice. Pour all over scallops.
- In another small bowl, combine bread crumbs, Parmesan, oil, and red pepper flakes. Sprinkle mixture on top of each scallop.
- Bake until tops are golden and scallops are translucent, 12 to 15 minutes.
- Spoon butter over tops and serve with lemon wedges.

# Day 27

## Breakfast

### Grilled Mediterranean Vegetable Salad

Preparation Time: 20 Mins
Cook Time: 15 Mins
Total Time: 35 Mins
Servings: 4-6
Ingredients

- 1 to 2 tablespoons olive oil, for brushing vegetables
- 1 onion (large sliced)
- 2 zucchini (large sliced)
- 2 bell peppers (red, seeded and quartered)
- 2 eggplants (medium sliced into 1/2-inch-thick rounds)
- 1 potato (large parboiled and sliced)
- Garnish: Feta cheese (crumbled for serving)

### For the Vinaigrette

- 5 tablespoons olive oil
- 1 garlic clove (peeled and smashed with the flat side of knife)
- 3 tablespoons balsamic vinegar
- 1 teaspoon mint (dried)
- 1 teaspoon oregano (dried)

### Pinch: Marjoram (Dried)

- 1/2 teaspoon salt (coarse)
- 1/4 teaspoon black pepper (freshly ground)

Instructions
- Gather the ingredients.
- Add the ingredients to a small bottle or bowl and shake or whisk together

- Allow the vinaigrette to sit for about 1/2 an hour for the flavors to meld
- Discard the garlic clove before using.
- Heat the grill to medium-high.
- Lightly brush the vegetables with olive oil and grill for about 5 minutes on each side or until tender.
- cut larger pieces into chunks and toss with dressing in a large bowl.
- Sprinkle with crumbled Feta cheese and serve immediately.
- Enjoy!

Nutrition per servings: 302 calories.

## Lunch

### Bibimbap

Preparation Time: 40 Mins
Cook Time: 30 Mins
Total 1hr 10 Mins
Servings: 4
Ingredients
- 4 cups cooked white rice , preferably short grain (note 1)
- 4 eggs
- 2 tsp sesame seeds
- 250 g/8oz beef tenderloin or thick steak , very finely sliced (subs, Note 2)
- 1/4 green apple , grated using box grater (Note 3)
- 3 garlic cloves , minced
- 1 tbsp soy sauce , light or all purpose (Note 4)
- 1 tbsp honey (or brown sugar)
- 2 tsp sesame oil , toasted (Note 9)

### Vegetable

- 2 carrots , large, cut into 5 x 0.5cm/2 x 1/5" batons
- 2 zucchini , large, cut into 5 x 0.5cm/2 x 1/5" batons
- 1 bunch of spinach , cut into 5cm/2" lengths

- 8 dried shiitake mushrooms , large (Note 5)
- 4 cups bean sprouts
- 2 tsp garlic , minced (3 cloves)
- 8 tsp vegetable oil , separated
- 1/2 tsp salt
- 1.5 tsp soy sauce , light or all purpose (Note 4)
- 1/4 tsp fish sauce (sub soy)
- 1/4 tsp white sugar
- Sesame oil , toasted (Note 9)

Bibimbap Sauce:

- 4 tbsp gochujang paste (Note 6)
- 2 tbsp mirin (Note 7)
- 2 tbsp rice vinegar (Note 8)
- 1.5 tsp soy sauce (Note 4)
- 3 tsp white sugar
- 1 garlic clove , finely grated
- 2.5 tsp sesame oil , toasted (Note 9)

Instructions

Bibimbap Sauce:

- Mix ingredients until sugar is dissolved.

Marinated Beef:

- Mix the marinade in a bowl, then add beef. Marinate for 30 minutes to overnight.
- Heat 2 tsp oil in a large skillet over high heat. Let excess marinade drip off then add beef. Cook for 3 - 4 minutes until cooked and there's some caramelised bits, then remove from skillet.
- Keep warm until required or reheat to warm.

Prepare Vegetables:

- Shiitake: Soak mushrooms in a large bowl of boiling water for 30 minutes, or until rehydrated. Drain, squeeze out excess water, then slice.
- Carrot and Zucchini salting (optional, Note 10): Place carrot and zucchini in separate bowls, sprinkle each with 1/4 tsp salt, toss, leave for 20 minutes then drain excess liquid.

## Cook Vegetables:

- Get 2 skillets going if you can!
- Shiitake: Heat 2 tsp oil oil in a skillet over medium high heat. Cook mushrooms for 2 minutes. Add 1.5 tsp soy, 1/4 tsp sugar, 1/2 tsp of garlic. Stir for 1 minute, then remove.
- Carrot: Add 2 tsp oil into the skillet, cook carrot until just tender (5 to 8 minutes), then remove.
- Zucchini: Cook as with carrot for 4 minutes.
- Spinach: Heat 2 tsp veg with a splash of sesame oil. Saute until starting to wilt. Add 1/2 tsp garlic, and salt to taste, stir, then remove. When cool, squeeze to drain out excess liquid.
- Beansprouts: Simmer in water for 5 min or steam in microwave for 3 min until floppy. Drain under cold water, then cool. Squeeze out excess liquid with hands, place in bowl. Mix with 2 tsp sesame oil, 1 tsp garlic, 1/4 tsp fish sauce.
- Vegetables can cool, they are meant to be at room temp or slightly warm.

## Assemble:

- Fry eggs in a skillet to your taste (I like mine with runny yolks).
- Place warm rice in bowls.
- Top with vegetables and beef, as pictured in post, then lastly, the egg.

- Sprinkle with sesame seeds, drizzled with sesame oil. Serve with Bibimbap Sauce!

# Dinner

## Seitan Curry

Preparation Time: 5 Mins
Cook Time: 15 Mins
Total Time: 20 Mins
Servings: 8
Ingredients
- 1 tablespoon coconut oil (or any vegetable oil)
- ½ recipe Indian curry paste
- 8 oz seitan crumbles
- 8 oz cremini mushrooms (or button mushrooms, portobello mushrooms, shiitake mushrooms or oyster mushrooms. You can also use wild dry mushrooms, reconstituted)
- ½ cup coconut milk
- 1 tablespoon kasoori methi (dry fenugreek leaves. Crush between your palms before adding to pot)
- 1 teaspoon sugar
- Salt to taste
- 3 scallions (trimmed, green and white parts chopped. Optional. You can also use cilantro.)

Instructions
- eat coconut oil in large pot or Dutch oven. Add curry paste. Mix well, cover, and let the curry paste cook 10 minutes over low heat, stirring fre?uently, until glossy.
- Add the mushrooms and seitan crumbles to the pot. Add 1 cup water, mix, and bring to a boil. Lower the heat and simmer for another five minutes to let the flavors incorporate.
- Stir in coconut milk and kasoori methi. Mix. Finally stir in the sugar and mix well. Add salt to taste and turn off heat. Garnish with scallions, if using, or with cilantro.

# Day 28

## Breakfast

Fluffy Pancakes

Preparation Time: 10 Mins
Cook Time: 20 Mins
Total Time: 30 Mins
Servings: 1
Ingredients
- 1 ½ cups (195 grams) all-purpose flour, see tips below for how to measure flour
- 2 tablespoons sugar
- 1 tablespoon aluminum-free baking powder, see notes for substituting baking soda
- 1/2 teaspoon of fine sea or table salt, reduce to 1/4 teaspoon if sensitive to salt
- 1 ¼ cups (295 ml) milk, dairy or non-dairy
- 1 large egg
- 4 tablespoons unsalted butter, melted, plus more for skillet
- 1 teaspoon vanilla extract

Instructions
- Make Batter
- Whisk flour, sugar, baking powder, and the salt in a medium bowl.
- Warm milk in the microwave or on top of the stove until lukewarm, not hot. You should be able to keep your finger submerged for 10 seconds.
- Whisk milk, egg, melted butter, and vanilla extract until combined. (By warming the milk slightly, the melted butter mixes into the milk instead of turning into small lumps).
- Cook pancakes
- Heat a large skillet (or use griddle) over medium heat. The pan is ready if when you splatter a little water onto the pan

surface, the water dances around the pan and eventually evaporates.

- Make a well in the center of the flour mixture, pour milk mixture into the well and use a fork to stir until you no longer see clumps of flour. It is okay if the batter has small lumps – it is important not to over-mix the batter.
- Lightly brush skillet with melted butter (this is optional if you have a high-quality non-stick pan). Use a 1/4-cup measuring cup to spoon batter onto the skillet. Gently spread the batter into a 4-inch circle.
- When edges look dry, and bubbles start to appear and pop on the top surfaces of the pancake, turn over. This takes about 2 minutes. Once flipped, cook another 1 to 2 minutes or until lightly browned and cooked in the middle. Serve immediately with warm syrup, butter, and berries.

# Lunch

## Seedy Muesli Bar Slice

Cooking Time: 25 Mins
Ingredients
- 1cup rolled oats
- 1cup desiccated coconut
- ½cup wheat germ or 1/2 cup wheat bran
- ½cup sesame seeds
- ½cup sunflower seeds
- ½cup pumpkin seeds (pepita)
- 1cup sultana
- 125g butter (1/2 cup)
- ½cup honey
- ⅓cup brown sugar

Instructions
- Grease and line 3cm deep 16 x 28cm baking pan with baking paper.

- Cook oats, coconut, wheatgerm, sesame seeds, sunflower kernels and pumpkin seeds in frying pan over med heat stirring 8-10 min until golden. Place in a large bowl to cool and stir in sultanas.
- Cook butter, honey and sugar over med heat, stirring, for 3-4 min until sugar dissolves. Reduce to low and simmer without stirring for 7 minute.
- Add to dry ingredients and mix well.
- Spoon into pan and press down firmly, allow to set for a few hours in the fridge, then cut into slices and enjoy!

## Dinner

No-Tuna Salad

Preparation Time: 10 Mins
Servings: 4
Ingredients

For the Salad:

- 1 (15-ounce) can chickpeas, rinsed and drained
- 3 tablespoons tahini
- 1 teaspoon Dijon or spicy brown mustard
- 1 tablespoon maple syrup or agave nectar
- ¼ cup diced red onion
- ¼ cup diced celery
- ¼ cup diced pickle
- 1 teaspoon capers, drained and loosely chopped
- Healthy pinch each sea salt and black pepper
- 1 tablespoon roasted unsalted sunflower seeds (optional)

For Serving:

- 8 slices whole-wheat bread
- Dijon or spicy brown mustard
- Romaine lettuce

- Tomato, sliced
- Red onion, sliced

Instructions

- Place the chickpeas in a mixing bowl and mash with a fork, leaving only a few beans whole.
- Add tahini, mustard, maple syrup, red onion, celery, pickle, capers, salt and pepper, and sunflower seeds (if using) to mixing bowl. Mix to incorporate. Taste and adjust seasonings as needed.
- Toast bread if desired, and prepare any other desired sandwich toppings (such as lettuce, tomato, and onion).
- Scoop a healthy amount of the chickpea mixture (about ½ cup) onto one slice of bread, add desired toppings and top with second slice of bread. Repeat for additional sandwiches.

# Day 29

## Breakfast

### Basic Pie Dough

Preparation Time: 10 Mins
Total Time: 2 Hrs 10 Mins
Ingredients
- 2 1/2 c. all-purpose flour, spooned and leveled
- 1 tsp. Kosher salt
- 1 tsp. sugar
- 1 c. cold unsalted butter, cut up
- 1/4 c. ice water

Instructions
- Whisk together flour, salt, and sugar. Cut in butter until it resembles coarse meal with several pea-size pieces remaining. Add water, 1 tablespoon at a time, using a fork to pull dough together into a crumbly pile (add up to an additional 2 tablespoons of water if needed).
- Divided dough into two piles; wrap each in plastic wrap. Use the plastic to flatten and press dough into disks. Refrigerate until firm, 2 hours.
- Bring dough to room temperature and roll out on a counter or cutting board lightly dusted with flour until 1/8 inch thick. Then press into pan and par-bake or fill as pie recipe instructs.

## Lunch

### Bavarian Beef

Preparation time: 8 hrs 30 mins
Servings: 6-8
Ingredients
- 2 -3lbs boneless beef chuck roast
- 1tablespoon cooking oil

- 2cups sliced carrots
- 3/4cup chopped kosher dill pickle
- 1cup sliced celery
- 1/2cup dry red wine or 1/2 cup beef broth
- 1/3cup German mustard
- 1/2teaspoon fresh coarse ground black pepper
- 1/4teaspoon ground cloves
- 2bay leaves
- 2tablespoons flour
- 2tablespoons dry red wine or 2 tablespoons beef broth
- hot cooked noodles
- chopped dill pickle (garnish)
- cooked crumbled bacon (garnish)
- 1large onion, sliced

## Instructions

- Trim fat from roast.
- In a large skillet, brown roast on all sides in hot oil.
- Meanwhile in place carrots, onions, 3/4 pickles, and celery in crock pot.
- Place meat on top of veggies, cutting the roast to fit, if necessary.
- In a small bowl, combine wine or broth, mustard, pepper, cloves and bay leaves.
- Pour over meat.
- Cover and cook on LOW for 8 to 10 hours; or HIGH for 4 to 5 hours.
- Remove meat from pot and place on platter, keeping warm.
- For gravy: transfer the cooking liquid to a 2 Quart saucepan.
- Skim off fat and remove bay leaves.
- Stir together the flour and the remaining 2 tablespoons wine or broth.
- Stir into the gravy mixture.
- Cook and stir over medium heat until thickened an bubbly.
- Add vegetables and stir one or two more minutes more to warm up vegetables.

- Serve the meat with vegetable gravy and noodles.
- Garnish with chopped pickles and bacon.

## Dinner

### Berry Sauce

Preparation Time: 10 Minutes
Cook Time: 10 Mins
Total Time: 20 Minutes
Servings: 8-10
Ingredients
- 1 lb fresh strawberries, hulled and thinly sliced
- 6 oz (1 dry half pint) fresh raspberries
- 6 oz (1 dry half pint) fresh blueberries
- 6 oz (1 dry half pint) fresh blackberries
- 1 tablespoon fresh lemon juice, from 1 lemon
- ¾ cup sugar

Instructions
- Combine all of the berries in a large bowl and stir gently to combine. Spoon about ⅔ of the mixed berries into a medium saucepan; transfer the remaining berries to a small bowl and refrigerate until ready to serve.
- Add the lemon juice and sugar to the berries in the sauce pan. Bring to a gentle boil over medium heat and cook until the fruit is syrupy, about 5 minutes.
- Transfer the hot berry mixture to a blender and purée until smooth. Set a fine mesh strainer over a bowl. Pour the sauce into the strainer and use the back of a soup ladle and circular motions to force the sauce through the strainer and into the bowl. Discard the seeds that remain in the strainer. Refrigerate the berry sauce until cold or ready to serve.
- Before serving, add the reserved berries to the sauce and stir to combine. If the sauce seems too thick, add a few tablespoons of water, a little at a time, until the desired consistency is reached.

# Day 30

Breakfast
Preparation Time: 5 Minutes
Cook Time: 20 Minutes
Total Time: 25 Minutes
Ingredients
- 1 large sweet potato
- 5 eggs
- 1/2 cup chopped spinach
- 1/2 of an onion
- 1/4-1/2 cup feta cheese
- Salt
- Olive oil
- Pepper
- I added 1/2 tsp Chipotle powder to give them a little spice!

Instructions
- Preheat oven to 400F
- Using a cheese grater, cut the sweet potato into smaller pieces. 3. Take a towel and squeeze the extra moisture from the sweet potatoes. Then add to a bowl and add 1 tsp olive oil and coat the sweet potato
- Then either use muffin liners or grease a muffin tin well.
- Line 12 cups about halfway with the sweet potato, patting it down
- Bake for 10 minutes
- While that bakes, sauté your onion for 4-5 minutes in some olive oil
- Then add in spinach and saute´ another 1-2 minutes
- Crack eggs into a bowl and whisk.
- Then add in the saute´ed veggies + feta
- Mix together well, sprinkle some salt & pepper in here
- When the sweet potato part is done, remove and pour the egg mixture on top.
- Return to oven and bake another 12-13 minutes (until the egg is hardened)

- Remove and let cool before removing
- Store about 4-5 days in the fridge! Makes 12 cups.

# Lunch

## Mackerel Pate

Prep Time: 30 Mins
Servings: 6
Ingredients
- 1 pack smoked mackerel (about 200g)
- 250g tub cream cheese
- 2 lemons, 1 zested, both juiced
- small pack dill, half roughly chopped, half fronds picked
- 1 cucumber
- 4 tbsp olive oil, plus extra to drizzle

Instructions
- Peel and flake the mackerel and tip into a small blender with the cream cheese, lemon zest and half the lemon juice, and pulse to make a pâté. Add the chopped dill and pulse again to mix.
- Tip the mixture into a plastic piping bag or sandwich bag, cut off the end and pipe six thick cylinders of the pâté onto a baking tray and put in the freezer to harden for about 1 hr.
- Remove a strip of peel from the cucumber – it's easiest with a swivel peeler, but a normal one also works – then peel 12 neat ribbons off the cucumber. Do not throw away any of the seeds or the peelings. Dice any remaining flesh, cover and put in the fridge ready to use later. Use the neat ribbons to wrap around the pâté and put in the fridge. Can be made up to 1 day ahead.
- Tip the cucumber peelings and seeds into a blender or smoothie maker with the rest of the lemon juice, the olive oil and some seasoning. Blitz to make a thick dressing, then chill. Can be made 1 day ahead and kept in the fridge.

- To serve, pour a little dressing onto each plate, sit a cucumber-wrapped pâté on top, neatly scatter the diced cucumber and dill fronds, and drizzle over more olive oil.

# Dinner

## Hummus

Cook Time: 20 Mins
Preparation Time: 20 Mins
Total Time: 40 Mins
Servings: 8
Ingredients
- 1 can (15 ounces) chickpeas, rinsed and drained, or 1 ½ cups cooked chickpeas
- ½ teaspoon baking soda (if you're using canned chickpeas)
- ¼ cup lemon juice (from 1 ½ to 2 lemons), more to taste
- 1 medium-to-large clove garlic, roughly chopped
- ½ teaspoon fine sea salt, to taste
- ½ cup tahini
- 2 to 4 tablespoons ice water, more as needed
- ½ teaspoon ground cumin
- 1 tablespoon extra-virgin olive oil
- Any of the following garnishes: drizzle of olive oil or zhoug sauce, sprinkle of ground sumac or paprika, chopped fresh parsley

Instructions
- Place the chickpeas in a medium saucepan and add the baking soda. Cover the chickpeas by several inches of water, then bring the mixture to a boil over high heat. Continue boiling, reducing heat if necessary to prevent overflow, for about 20 minutes, or until the chickpeas look bloated, their skins are falling off, and they're quite soft. In a fine-mesh strainer, drain the chickpeas and run cool water over them for about 30 seconds. Set aside (no need to peel the chickpeas for this recipe!).

- Meanwhile, in a food processor or high-powered blender, combine the lemon juice, garlic and salt. Process until the garlic is very finely chopped, then let the mixture rest so the garlic flavor can mellow, ideally 10 minutes or longer.
- Add the tahini to the food processor and blend until the mixture is thick and creamy, stopping to scrape down any tahini stuck to the sides and bottom of the processor as necessary.
- While running the food processor, drizzle in 2 tablespoons ice water. Scrape down the food processor, and blend until the mixture is ultra smooth, pale and creamy. (If your tahini was extra-thick to begin with, you might need to add 1 to 2 tablespoons more ice water.)
- Add the cumin and the drained, over-cooked chickpeas to the food processor. While blending, drizzle in the olive oil. Blend until the mixture is super smooth, scraping down the sides of the processor as necessary, about 2 minutes. Add more ice water by the tablespoon if necessary to achieve a super creamy texture.
- Taste, and adjust as necessary—I almost always add another ¼ teaspoon salt for more overall flavor and another tablespoon of lemon juice for extra zing.
- Scrape the hummus into a serving bowl or platter, and use a spoon to create nice swooshes on top. Top with garnishes of your choice, and serve. Leftover hummus keeps well in the refrigerator, covered, for up to 1 week.

Printed in Great Britain
by Amazon

45520416R00066